S. Riaskoff

DIABETIC RETINOPATHY

Dr. W. Junk bv Publishers 1976

2

ISBN-13: 978-90-6193-554-4   e-ISBN-13: 978-94-010-1581-3
DOI: 10.1007/978-94-010-1581-3
© Dr. W. Junk bv Publishers The Hague
Lay-out and coverdesign: Max Velthuijs

Contents

4

Introduction

The evaluation of diabetic retinopathy is often difficult, because the clinical picture is complex due to the multiplicity of symptoms. Omission of treatment by photocoagulation at the right moment may have grave consequences.

For the evaluation of diabetic retinopathy we have to estimate first the developmental degree of each symptom and secondly we have to estimate what the natural history of each particular retinopathy will be.
There exists a number of classification systems, into the frame of which the clinical picture of diabetic retinopathy can be placed. Without entering into the details of these systems we want to mention that our classification has been developed from the method of Oakley and the classification model conceived at the Airlie House meeting in 1968.
The essence of this classification is that standard pictures are used for the estimation of the developmental degree of the different symptoms in diabetic retinopathy.
In our classification we use for each symptom two standard photographs instead of one, as originally proposed at the Airlie House meeting. (1, 2).
Standard photograph number one stands for the moderate (grade 1) manifestation and standard photograph number two stands for the marked (grade 2) manifestation of the symptom.
If the manifestation of the sympton is less marked than in standard photograph one, it is referred to as <1 ; if it is more marked than in standard photograph two, it is referred to as >2.

We are presenting here a collection of fundus photographs which in our experience can serve as examples of the moderate and of the marked manifestation of the symptoms of diabetic retinopathy. The aim of this collection is to provide pictures for the use by the ophthalmologist, who is confronted with the problems of diabetic retinopathy, but lacks the experience needed for the correct management of these problems.
It should help him to evaluate properly the clinical picture presented by his patient by comparing the fundus picture with the fundus photographs with the aim of predicting the future development of the retinopathy.
For this purpose the stage of development of diabetic retinopathy presented in the different examples is described and a prognosis is made. Special attention is paid to the prognostic value of the different symptoms of diabetic retinopathy.

Stage I:
Early diabetic retinopathy.
The symptoms are still moderate. The prediction of further development is difficult. Prognosis is still good or uncertain.

Stage II:
Advanced diabetic retinopathy.
The symptoms are clearly marked. A further progression of the diabetic retinopathy seems very probable. Visual acuity is still good, but is threatened by deterioration. Prognosis is serious.

Stage III:

Very advanced diabetic retinopathy.
The symptoms are widespread and strongly marked. Visual acuity is affected. Further
progression to social or total blindness is probable.
Prognosis is poor.

Stage IV:
The final stage of diabetic retinopathy.
The disease has reached the terminal stage. To this stage belong: massive intravitreal
haemorrhages without tendency to resorption, detachment of the retina, and
haemorrhagic glaucoma.
Prognosis is in these cases mostly hopeless. There are, however, cases in which
some visual function is retained (sometimes about 1–2/60) and the evolution to
total blindness does not occur. This may be due to spontaneously stabilized
proliferative diabetic retinopathy with widespread avascular strands and very
advanced arterial obliteration without retinal detachment.

We avoided in this classification qualifying the clinical picture by benign or simple
on the one hand and proliferative, or severe on the other. A non-proliferative diabetic
retinopathy with massive lipoid deposits in the macular area and a visual acuity
which is approaching blindness should be regarded as a very advanced stage III
retinopathy. It cannot receive the adjective benign or simple only on account of
lack of proliferative changes. In our opinion it is therefore better to classify diabetic
retinopathy not on the basis of existing or non-existing proliferative changes, but
on the basis of the clinical appearance as a whole. Nevertheless after having classified
the clinical picture, if there is neovascularization or any other proliferative sign,
we should notice it because of its importance for the further evolution and the
prognosis. Examples of our classification method are given in the table after the
series of fundus photographs.

The training in correct evaluation of diabetic retinopathy becomes more and more
important nowadays because the indication to treat a case with light-coagulation
mainly depends on it. Besides this we would like to stress the importance of predicting
what we can expect of light-coagulation treatment in each particular case. We
should be able to state in advance what we expect to achieve by this treatment
and what we cannot expect to.
In order to procure information about the effect of light-coagulation treatment we
have included in the text and in the series of fundus photographs some of our
observations over a 6-year follow-up period. In each case details about the extent
of treatment and a comment on its results are given.
We intentionally do not discuss the results which are supplied by more sophisticated
investigations as fluorescein angiography and electro-diagnostic tests.

Our intention is to present the clinical appearance of diabetic retinopathy and the
possible influence of photocoagulation treatment on its course in a simple but
more or less complete series of fundus pictures comparable to those seen by the
ophthalmologist in his consulting room. We hope that by these means the
ophthalmologist can be helped in interpreting his findings and in advising his patients
as to the best moment to start treatment.

Evaluation of symptoms in diabetic retinopathy in relation to prognosis
and treatment with photocoagulation
Standard photographs

1 Microaneurysms (ma) and intraretinal haemorrhages (h)

Fig. 1 and 2: ma$_1$ h$_1$

Women, 24 years old, diabetes for 14 years. Left eye:
A few microaneurysms and intraretinal haemorrhages spread around the macula
and the optic disc are characteristic of moderate (grade 1) presentation of these
symptoms.
The arteries seem normal, the veins appear swollen but no beading is seen. Dilated
capillaries near arrows 1, old cotton wool patch near arrow 2. The macula is not
affected. Visual acuity: 1.0.

Stage I, early diabetic retinopathy.

Prognosis: good to doubtful. The doubtfulness is due to the fact that there are
swollen veins, dilated capillaries and old cotton wool patches. These signs point
to a decompensated circulation. Development of new vessels is to be expected.

Photocoagulation: treatment is indicated. However, if regular examination of the
patient every 3 months can be assured, treatment may be postponed. If progression
is seen it is advisable to start coagulation without delay.

Comment: The untreated left eye (fig. 1) has been followed for 3 years. The
right eye (fig. 3) of the same patient was treated at once. During the subsequent
period there was convincing evidence that treatment was beneficial (see fig. 3b)
while widespread neovascularization appeared in the untreated left eye. Extensive
photocoagulation of this eye could stop further evolution.
Visual acuity: OS=1.0 (2 years after treatment).

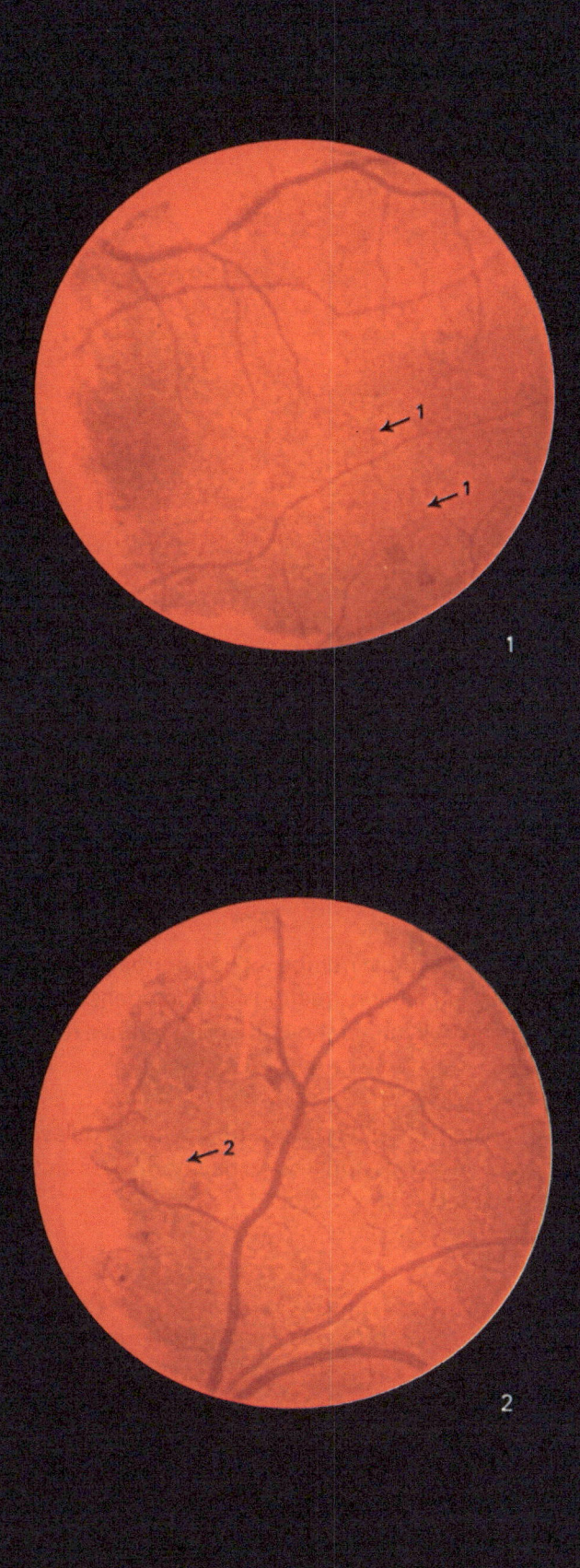

1

2

Fig. 3a: ma$_2$ h$_2$

Same patient. Right eye:
A great number of microaneurysms and intraretinal haemorrhages around the macular area, the disc and in the periphery of the retina are characteristic of marked (grade 2) presentation of these symptoms. Arteries and arterial branches appear normal. Veins are choked. Visual acuity: 1.0.

Stage II, advanced diabetic retinopathy.

Prognosis: uncertain to serious. A great number of haemorrhages, and a marked swelling of the veins show that circulation is seriously decompensated. Spontaneous improvement cannot be expected. Evolution toward a proliferative retinopathy is very likely.

Photocoagulation: is indicated. It is advisable to treat without delay. In this case widespread photocoagulation was applied. All haemorrhages and microaneurysms were coagulated (290 $\times$; spot 3°).

Fig. 3b

One year after photocoagulation haemorrhages and microaneurysms have completely disappeared.

Comment: This eye has been followed for more than 5 years. Visual acuity remained 0.9. No further treatment seemed necessary. However after a period of 5 years during which the clinical picture seemed stabilized and quiet, a preretinal haemorrhage occurred. The source was a small tuft of newly-formed vessels which had been obviously overlooked at the previous examination. This case demonstrates the importance of careful control examinations and repeated coagulation when progression is found.

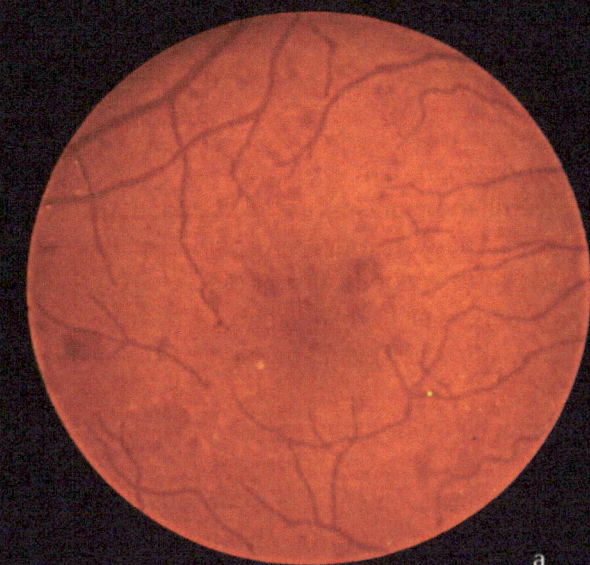

3

a

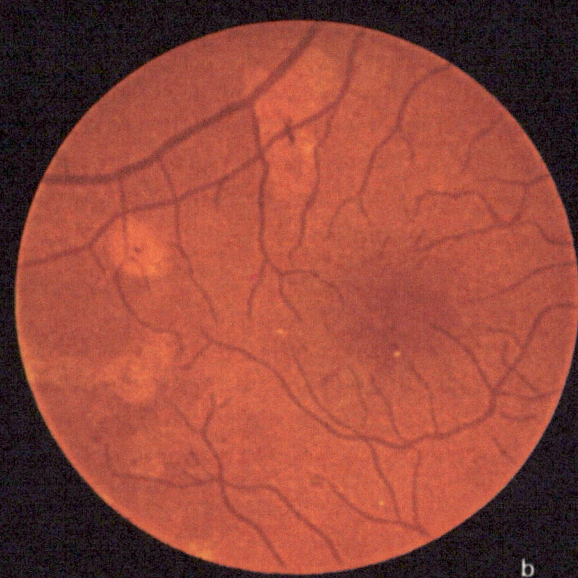

b

Fig. 4a: ma > 2 min h > 2 min

Man, 27 years old, diabetes for 15 years. Left eye:
Intraretinal haemorrhages and microaneurysms are so abundant that we should
grade this picture as ma > 2, h > 2. There are only a few hard exudates. Near the
temporal superior vein two old cotton-wool sports are seen (arrows). The arteries
are narrowed. The temporal superior vein is dilated and an initial beading pattern
is seen. The macula is severely affected. Visual acuity: 3/60.

Stage III: Very advanced diabetic retinopathy.

Prognosis: Poor. Spontaneous improvement seems most unlikely. It is very probable
that neovascularization will develop in the further evolution of the disease.

Photocoagulation: Treatment is strongly advised. Success, however, is uncertain.
Visual acuity is unlikely to improve but progression of retinopathy may be hold
back. If neovascularization is going to develop, it may be not so widespread as
without photocoagulation. In this case haemorrhages and microaneurysms all over
the fundus were coagulated (153 x 3° spot). Six months later a second treatment
was carried out (97 x, 4.5° spot).

Fig. 4b

One year after the first photocoagulation. Haemorrhages are less numerous; the
macular area however, is obviously not improved. Inferiorly to the macula an
obliterated arterial branch is seen (arrow 1). Dilated capillaries (arrows 2) give
evidence that neovascularization is setting in.

Fig. 4c

Two years after photocoagulation. Intraretinal haemorrhages are further diminished,
but more arterial branches are occluded (arrows), lipoid deposits have become
larger, and loops of new vessels have developed next the temporal superior vein (n.v.).
Visual acuity: 0.1.

Comment: The condition of the macular area remained poor and neovascularization
developed, despite widespread photocoagulation. Nevertheless the treatment should
not be judged as useless because the periphery of the retina became quiet, the
neovascularization kept confined to small areas and, as the follow up of one more
year proved, no complications occurred. Visual acuity did not deteriorate further.
Three years after photocoagulation vision was still 0.1. The right eye with the
same degree of diabetic changes was treated in the same way and was also stabilized.
Three years after photocoagulation visual acuity of the right eye was: 0.4.

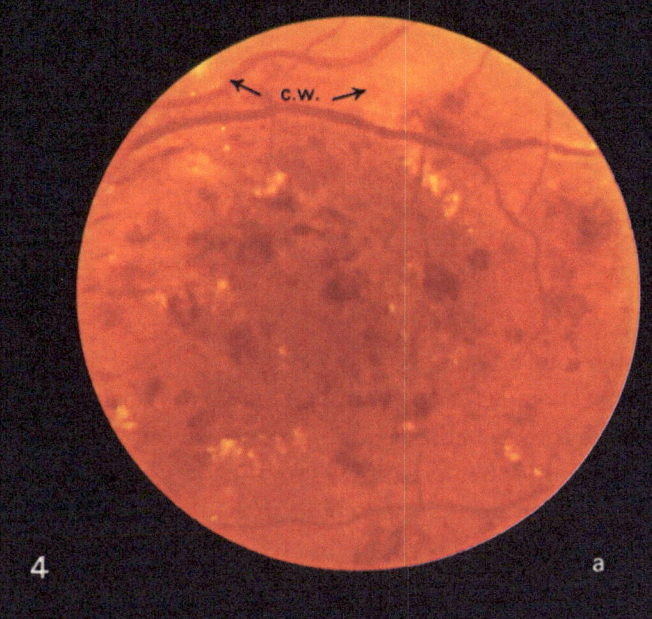

4

a

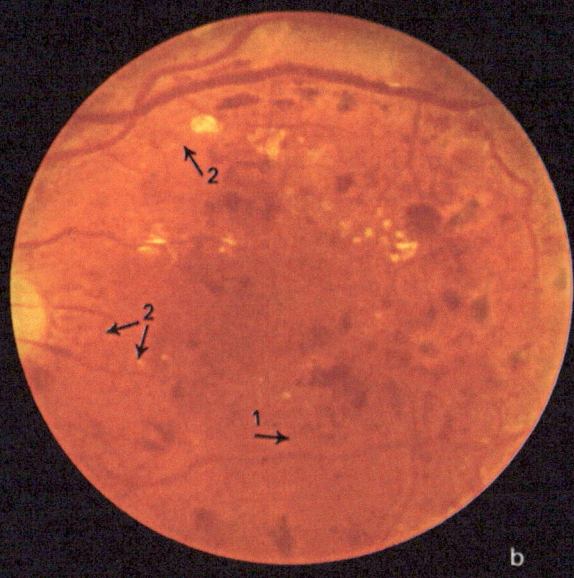

b

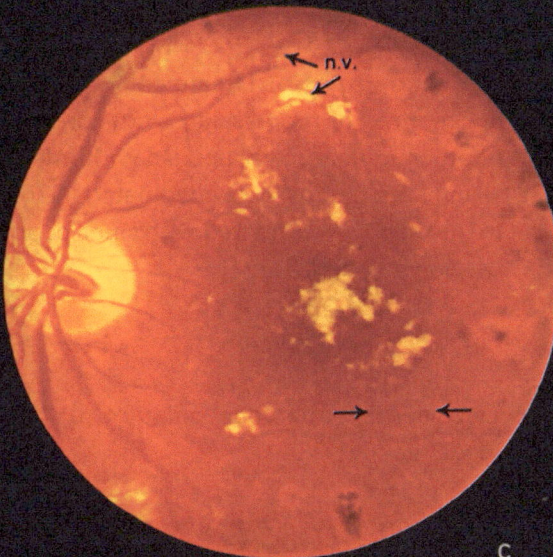

c

2 Lipoid deposits or hard exudates (e)

Fig. 5a: e_1

Man, 40 years old, diabetes for 15 years. Left eye:
A few lipoid deposits, mostly spread over the temporal part of the posterior pole
are characteristic of moderate (grade 1) hard exudates. The exudates are of small
size and are localized near and around microaneurysms and intraretinal haemorrhages.
The arteries appear normal. The temporal superior vein presents discrete irregularities
of the vessel wall. The macula seems to be normal but the microaneurysms in
this area prove that the capillary network around the macula is already damaged.
Visual acuity: 0.6.

Stage I–II, early diabetic retinopathy.

Prognosis: good or doubtful. The uncertainty of our prediction is due to the
fact that the macular area is already involved. Otherwise the non-progressive
appearance of this retinopathy would allow for a better prognosis.

Photocoagulation: treatment is indicated. However, it can be postponed for 3
or 6 months, as progression is not conspicuous. In this particular case
photocoagulation was applied without delay. Haemorrhages and microaneurysms
all over the fundus were coagulated (126 ×, 3° and 2° spot). The area temporal
to the macula was treated with small coagulation spots of low intensity as can
be viewed in Fig. 5b.

Fig. 5c

Two years after photocoagulation, exudates and haemorrhages have disappeared.
Visual acuity: 0.5.

Comment: Three years after the first photocoagulation a second treatment was
carried out (74 ×, 3°spot), since then during two more years of follow up, no
visible progression of the retinopathy was observed. Five years after treatment visual
acuity was 0.3. This slow deterioration of visual acuity is explained by the progression
of capillary occlusion around the macula, on which photocoagulation obviously has
no influence.
The right eye with an early diabetic retinopathy was left untreated for as long
as 4 years, when progression of lesions made photocoagulation necessary.
Visual acuity the year after treatment was: 0.7.

5

a

b

c

Fig. 6a: e₂

Woman, 50 years old, diabetes for 3 years. Right eye:
Numerous lipoid deposits, predominantly localized around microaneurysms and
intraretinal haemorrhages, and along the retinal vessels, are characteristic of marked
(grade 2) lipoid exudation.
In this case the ring of lipoid exudates is passing through the macular area. Inside
the ring microaneurysms and small intraretinal haemorrhages are seen. The temporal
superior vein is swollen with irregular walls (arrow 1). The artery crossing this
vein is also presenting some irregularities of the vessel wall (arrow 2).
Visual acuity: 0.3.

Stage II, advanced diabetic retinopathy.

Prognosis: doubtful, spontaneous improvement seems unlikely. The poor condition
of arteries and veins predicts further evolution toward neovascularization.

Photocoagulation: treatment is indicated. Postponing is not advisable on account
of possible rapid progression. In this case microaneurysms, intraretinal haemorrhages
and some small foci of neovascularization were treated (155×, 3°).

Fig. 6b

9 Months after photocoagulation. Retinopathy seems stabilized. Lipoid deposits
and foci of neovascularization disappeared.

Comment: Photocoagulation had a positive influence on exudative changes and
neovascularization. Visual acuity improved to 0.8. The patient has been under control
for 4 years after treatment. Neovascularization developed in the untreated left eye
and made photocoagulation necessary about 3 years after the treatment of the
right eye.

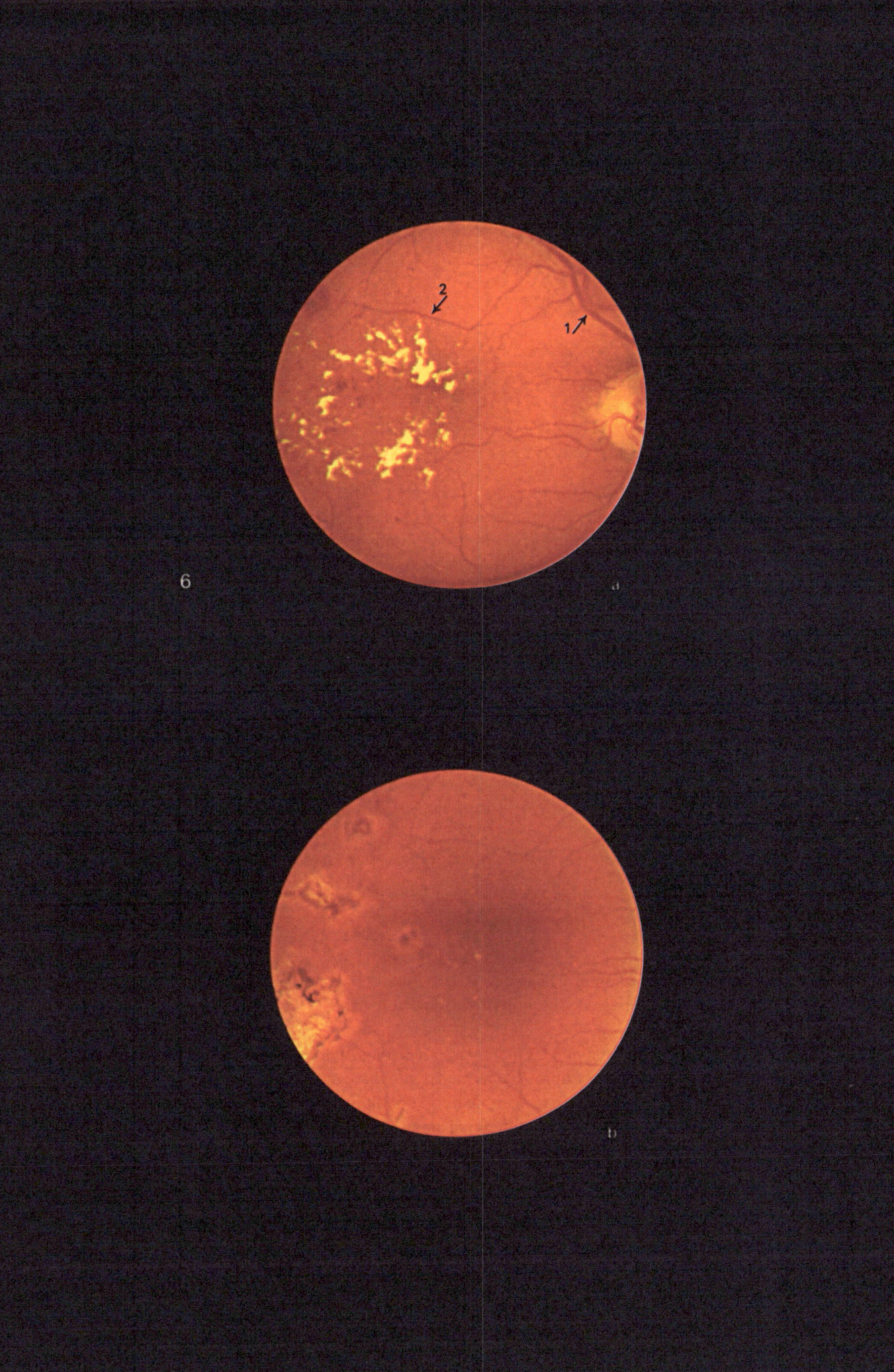

6

18

Fig. 7a: e>2

Woman, 52 years old, diabetes for 11 years. Right eye:
In this case the exudates were very numerous, with massive deposits at the posterior
pole and sheaths along some of the veins (arrows). Many intraretinal haemorrhages
were spread about the whole fundus, the arterial branches were narrowed but
not occluded. Visual acuity: 0.05.

Stage III, very advanced diabetic retinopathy.

Prognosis: poor. An increase of lipoid exudation is very likely. Neovascularization
may also develop in the further evolution of the disease.

Photocoagulation: treatment is indicated. It may stimulate the resorption of lipoid
deposits, prevent new exudative changes and neovascularization. If poor macular
function is partly due to oedema, an improvement of visual acuity may be expected
too.
In this case an extensive treatment of the whole fundus was carried out
(about 260 × , 4.5° spot).

Fig. 7b

One year after light-coagulation. The exudates and intraretinal haemorrhages have
almost completely disappeared. Retinopathy seems stabilized.

Comment: The condition remained quiet for about 6 years after treatment and
5 years after the photograph of figure 7b was made. The favorable effect of
photocoagulation is possibly due to the rather good condition of the retinal vessels.
By means of fluorescein angiography only small areas of capillary occlusion at
the posterior pole could be found. It is likely that the elimination of the pathologic
areas in the capillary network in the periphery of the retina led to an improvement
of blood circulation at the posterior pole which ensued resorption of lipoid deposits.
Visual acuity improved to 0.1 and remained so during the observation period. The
left eye which was not so seriously affected was treated also with a beneficial
effect. Visual acuity improved from 0.6 to 0.9 and remained so during the observation
period.

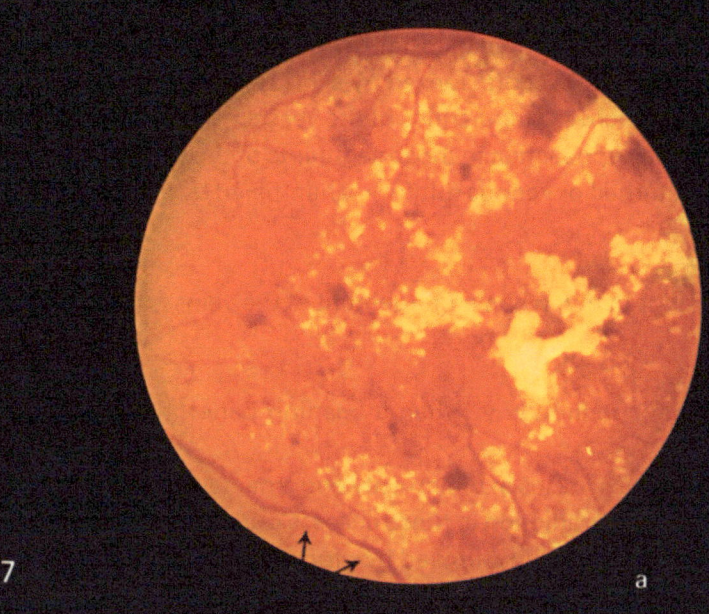

7

a

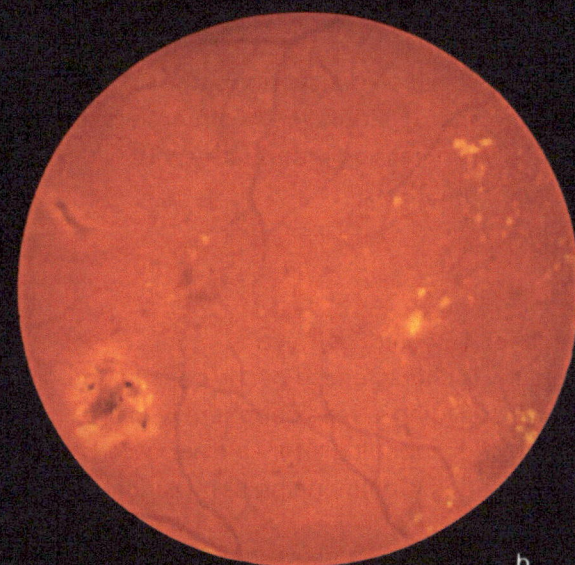

b

3 Changes of the veins (V) — diabetic venopathy

Fig. 8: V₁

Woman, 29 years old, diabetes for 19 years. Right eye:
The moderate diabetic venopathy is characterized by a diffuse engorgement of
the retinal veins and their branches. Irregularities of the vessel wall mark the further
evolution of venopathy. They appear first in those segments of the veins in which
arterial blood supply is disturbed or venous outflow is hampered by a crossing
artery.

Stage I, early diabetic retinopathy, when engorgement of the veins is the only
symptom.

Stage II, advanced diabetic retinopathy, when a beading pattern is seen.

Prognosis: good or doubtful in cases in which only engorgement of veins is
present. The uncertainty of our prediction in these cases is due to the experience
that engorgement of veins is frequently followed by progression of retinopathy.
The prognosis is serious or poor in cases in which the beading sign is present.
Beading occurs only when blood supply from terminal arterioles is irreversibly
disturbed. It is a preliminary or accompanying symptom of neovascularization.

Photocoagulation: venous changes are important when we consider the necessity
of photocoagulation. The presence of venous engorgement and of venous beading
is a strong support for treatment. After photocoagulation one may expect reduction
or disappearance of the engorgement.

Comment: In this case of a stage I—II diabetic retinopathy without
neovascularization, a moderate photocoagulation treatment was carried out. In spite
of this, 16 months later a rapidly progressing retinopathy with widespread
neovascularization developed (fig. 23a).

Fig. 9: V₂

Man, 52 years old, diabetic for 12 years. Left eye:
The marked diabetic venopathy is characterized by the conspicuous irregularities
of the vessel wall. In this figure beading is seen peripherally to the arterio-venous
crossing. The branches of the corresponding artery are narrowed; one of these
branches (arrow 1) seems occluded. Commencing neovascularization (arrow 2).
Visual acuity: 0.2.

Stage III, very advanced retinopathy with neovascularization.

Prognosis: poor. The marked beading of this vein is a sign that arterial blood
supply is severely hampered. Neovascularization is setting in.

Photocoagulation: treatment is strongly advised. The result is, however, uncertain.
The circulation seems already irreversibly disturbed.

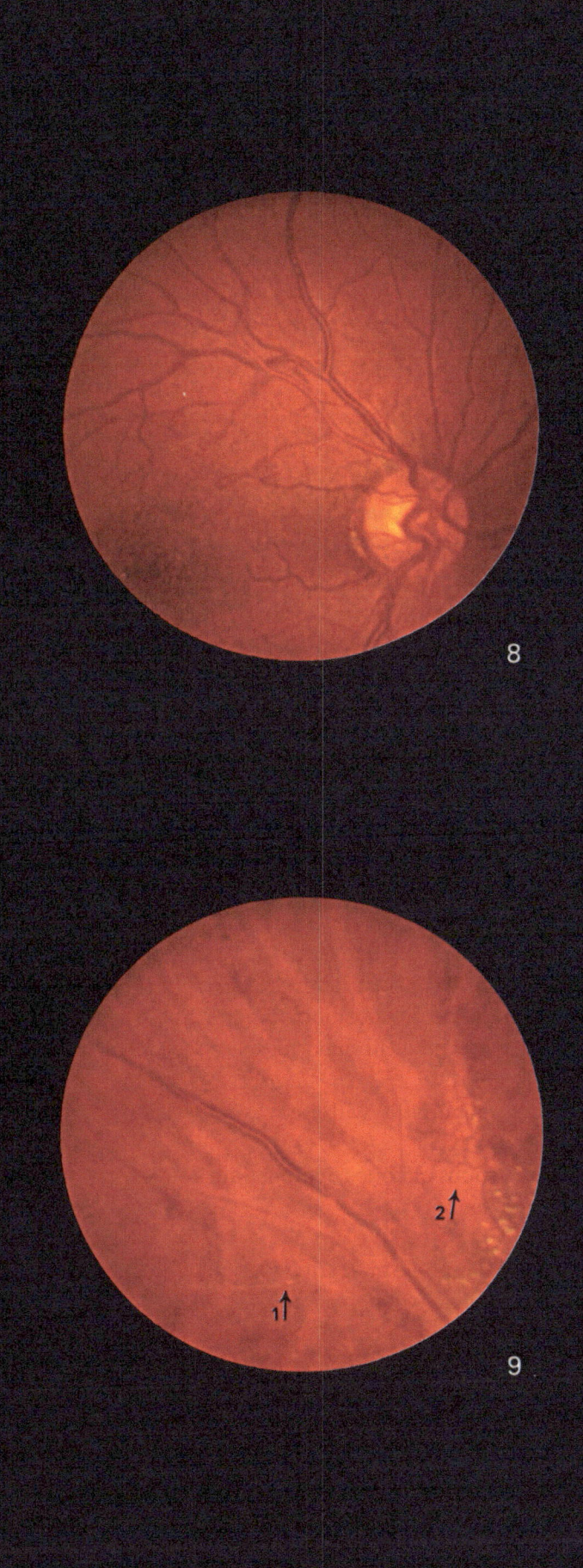

22

Comment: In this case only the right eye was treated. The left eye which is presented on fig. 9 was left untreated for comparison. Two years later visual acuity was OD = 0.1; OS = 1/60. Deterioration of visual acuity of the left eye was due to preretinal haemorrhages.

Fig. 10a, b; Fig. 11a, b: Evolution of moderate diabetic venopathy (V_1) to very marked venopathy ($V > 2$)

Man, 30 years old, diabetes for 12 years.
The very marked diabetic venopathy is characterized by the formation of venous collaterals and omega-like loops. As in venous engorgement and venous beading, these changes too depend on circulatory disturbances: influx deficiency from the corresponding arteries and reflux obstacles in the bypassed veins.

Fig. 10a presents the left eye before treatment with photocoagulation and fig. 10b the same eye 4 months after treatment
Fig. 11a presents the right eye before treatment with photocoagulation and fig. 11b the same eye $4\frac{1}{2}$ months after treatment.
On both photographs before treatment (fig. 10a and 11a) the arteries and their branches are not conspicuously pathologic. Faint cottonwool patches (cw), however, give evidence of occluded precapillary arterioles. Four months later some arteries are obviously narrowed (arrow 1) and others probably occluded (arrow 2).
The venous changes are more conspicuous too. Along the original vein a collateral vessel with many loops is found (fig. 10b, arrows 3). On fig. 11b along the venous branch running towards the 2 o'clock position numerous new vessel 'sprouts' are seen (arrows 4). Note also the fan of newly formed vessels above the disc (arrows 5).

Stage III, very advanced retinopathy with neovascularization.

Prognosis: poor. These venous changes demonstrate a severe and irreversible disturbance of retinal circulation.

Photocoagulation: the favourable effect of treatment with photocoagulation on retinal circulation is questionable when these severe venous changes are present. The indication to treatment should be considered on the basis of the other symptoms. The direct coagulation of collaterales and omega-loops is not advisable on account of possible ensuing haemorrhages. However the formation of scars next to those pathologic vessels could lead to reduction of leakage.

Comment: In this case, as in the case of fig. 8, photocoagulation was not able to stop the further evolution of diabetic retinopathy. The visual acuity of both eyes deteriorated within 2 years, the right eye becoming blind. Six years after treatment visual acuity was OD = Ø; OS = 0.25.

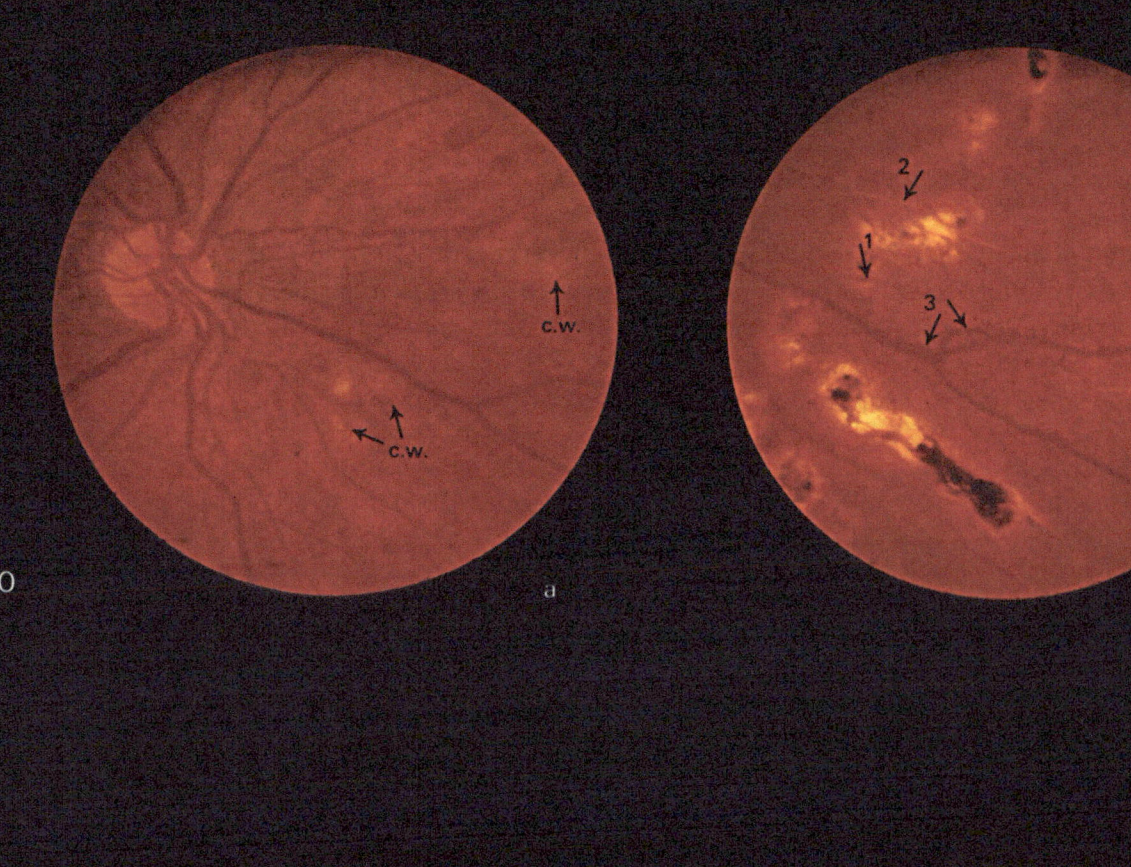

10

a

b

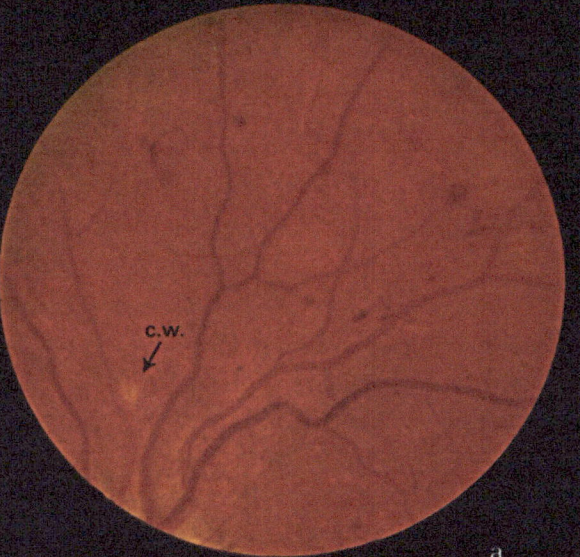

11

a

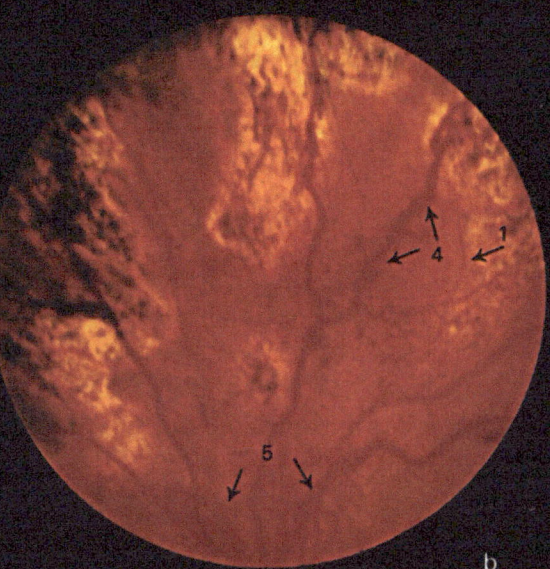

b

24

4 Changes of the arteries (A) — diabetic arteriolopathy

Fig. 12: A₁

Man, 48 years old, diabetes for 12 years. Right eye:

Fig. 13: A₁

Man, 51 years old, diabetes for 9 years. Left eye:

The moderate diabetic arteriolopathy is characterized by narrowing of the pre-terminal arterioles. The narrowing is more pronounced at the sites of their origin from the greater arterioles (arrows 1) and is often accompanied by irregularities of the vessel wall. Sometimes the narrowing is very marked so that the vessel is hardly seen (arrows 2; fig. 13). Visual acuity in the case of fig. 12: 0.4; in the case of fig. 13: 0.6.

Stage II, advanced diabetic retinopathy. These arteriolar changes are present in almost all cases of diabetic retinopathy with early neovascularization.

Prognosis: poor. Further progression is very likely. Spreading of neovascularization and degenerative changes in the macular area are expected if arterioles of this area are affected.

Photocoagulation: treatment is indicated in all cases in which neovascularization and widespread intraretinal haemorrhages are present. Photocoagulation has however no influence on the occlusive process in the retinal arterioles. In both patients photocoagulation of the peripheral changes was carried out with the Xenon arc while the changes at the posterior pole were treated with the Argon laser.

Comment: progression of the intraretinal haemorrhages, exudates and neovascularization could be stopped. The macular function did not improve. Two years after treatment the visual acuity was: in the case of fig. 12 = 0.3, in the case of fig. 13 = 0.4.

Fig. 14: A₂

Man, 22 years old, diabetes for 12 years. Left eye.
The marked arteriolopathy is characterized by the occlusion of the small arteriolar branches. In this case the arteriolar branches temporal to the macula are transformed into white threads (arrow 1); shunt vessels (arrow 2) and neovascularization (arrow 3) accompany the occlusive process. Visual acuity: 0.1.

Fig. 15: A₂

Woman, 70 years old, diabetes for 15 years. Right eye:
The peripheral part of an arterial branch is transformed into a white thread (arrow 1), occlusion of the next branch of the same artery is setting in (arrow 2), and marked neovascularization between both branches is present. Visual acuity: 0.1. The white thread appearance of an arterial branch should not be regarded as evidence of complete occlusion because on fluorography a slow bloodstream may be demonstrated in these arteries occasionally.

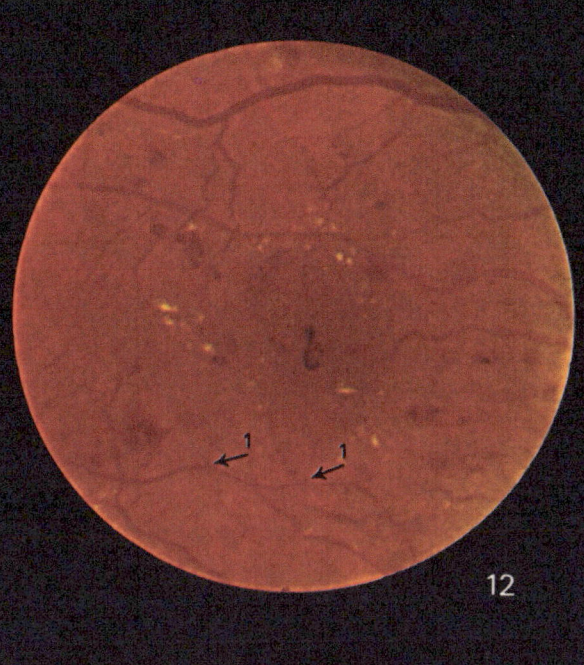

12

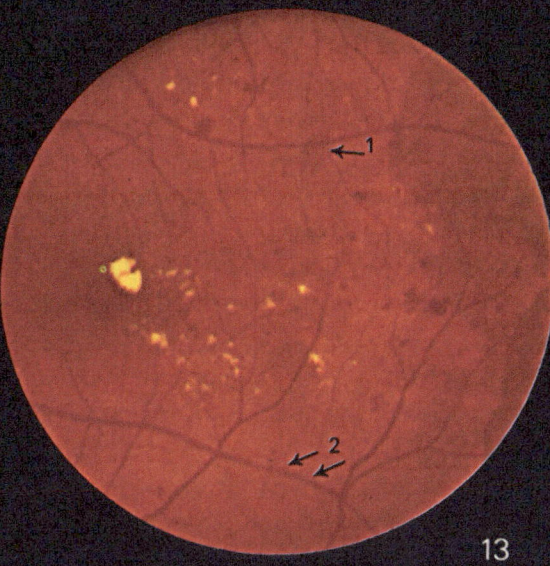

13

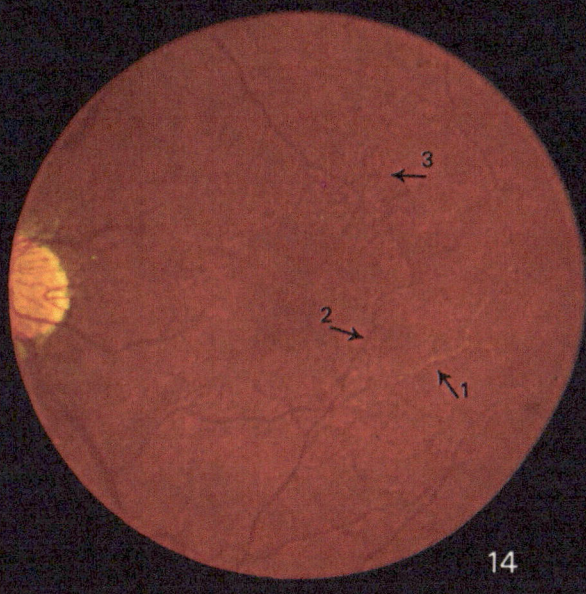

14

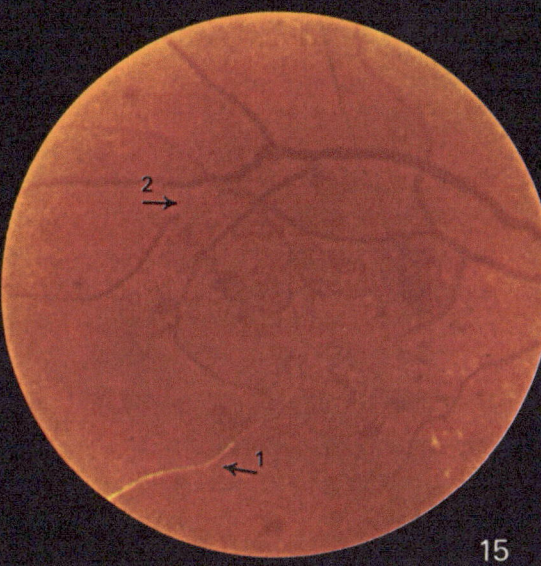

15

Stage III, very advanced diabetic retinopathy. The marked arteriolopathy with completely or almost completely occluded arterioles is a most important symptom of very advanced diabetic retinopathy with widespread neovascularization.

Prognosis: poor. The damage of the retina is extensive. Perimetry demonstrates wedge-shaped defects in the small isopters and irregular scotomas spread all over the central field. Electro-ophthalmological examination gives evidence of retinal hypoxia due to irreversible circulatory disturbance.
Nevertheless with progression of arteriolopathy the other symptoms of diabetic retinopathy often start a regressive course: intraretinal haemorrhages disappear, newly formed vessels become anaemic and are slowly obliterated.

Photocoagulation: treatment is indicated when neovascularization and haemorrhagic activity are still present.

Comment: the photocoagulation treatment was able to slow down and finally to stop neovascularization and probably to prevent massive haemorrhages. See also fig. 19, which presents a part of the fundus of the same eye as in fig. 14, before (a) and 1 year after treatment (b). Visual acuity which initially was 0.1 remained unchanged during the $3\frac{1}{2}$ years of follow-up.
The benefit of photocoagulation in this young man was unquestionable, because blindness within this period was very likely to occur without treatment. The second patient (fig. 15) died one year after photocoagulation.

5 Neovascularization of the retina (N)

Fig. 16: N_1

Woman, 24 years old, diabetes for 21 years; in the 8th month of pregnancy. Left eye:

The early neovascularization is characterized by the appearance of networks of dilated and hypertrophic capillary loops at the level of the retina. On this figure a number of cotton-wool patches are seen too. The branches of the artery which is running from left to right are conspicuously narrowed (arrows 1), the vein is somewhat dilated (arrow 2). Proximally to the arterio-venous crossing and in the area under the artery there is early neovascularization (arrow 3). Distally to the crossing site moderate beading of the vein can be observed (arrow 4).

Stage II–III, advanced diabetic retinopathy with early neovascularization.

Prognosis: serious. Retinal circulation is severely decompensated. Rapid progression of neovascularization is very likely.

Photocoagulation: treatment is strongly advised. By eliminating the newly-formed vessels and by the subsequent cicatrization of the corresponding areas of the retina one may expect firstly that the progression of the proliferative changes will be held back, and secondly that the blood stream will be led away from the more affected to the less affected areas of the vascular network. This last effect may be important as a means to preserve function of at least a part of the retina for a long period of time.

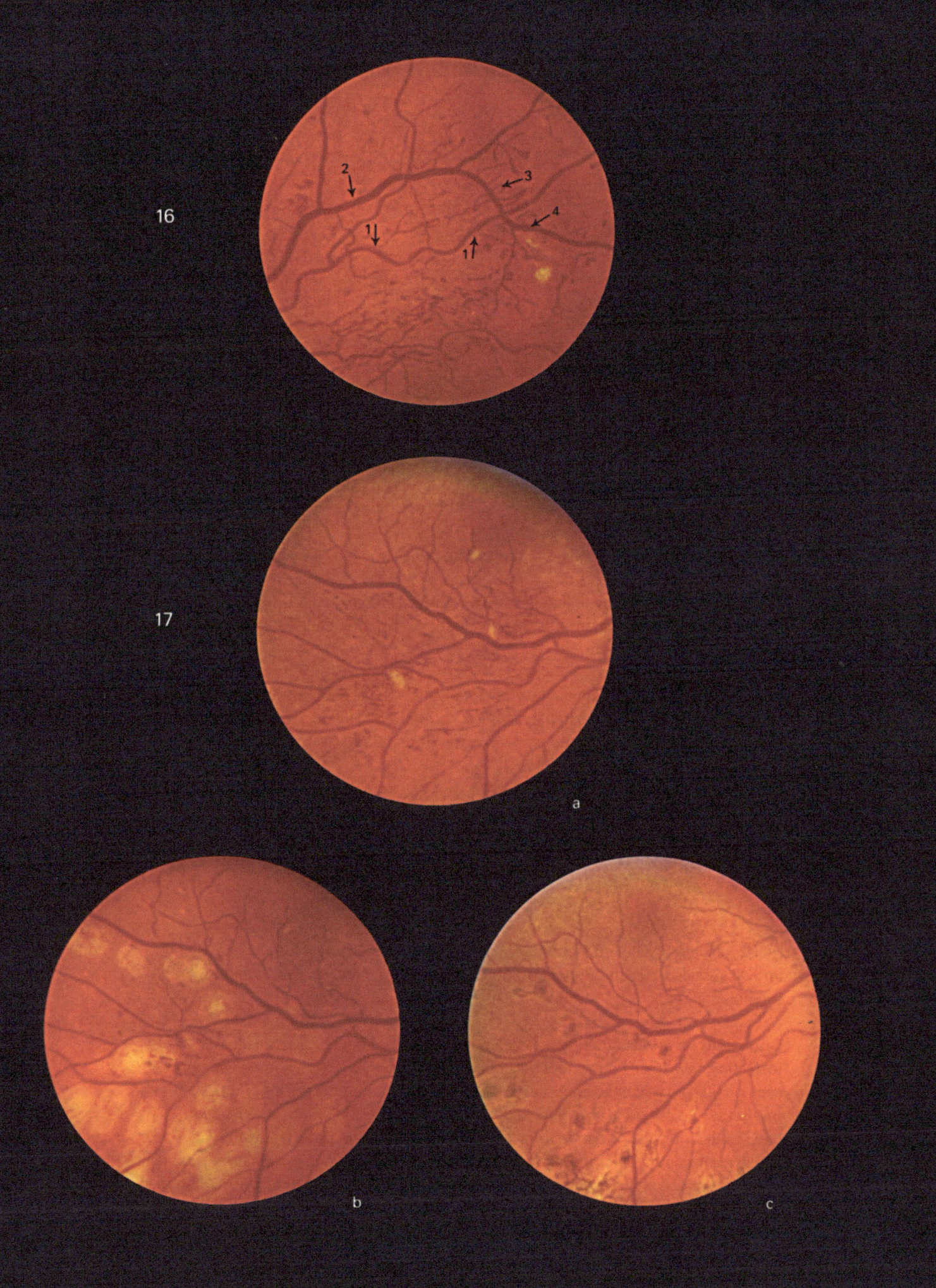

Fig. 17

Right eye of the same patient: a) before photocoagulation; b) one the day following treatment; c) 2 months later.

Comment: in the interval of two months, the birth took place. The retinopathy of the treated eye showed no progression, while the retinopathy of the untreated eye showed definite progression.

Fig. 18: N_2

Man, 26 years old, diabetes for 24 years. Right eye:

The marked neovascularization is characterized by the appearance of networks or 'fans' of newly-formed vessels of large calibre on the surface of the retina as seen in fig. 18a (arrow). Visual acuity: 1.0.

Stage III, very advanced diabetic retinopathy with marked neovascularization.

Prognosis: poor. However, in this case massive preretinal haemorrhages were not yet expected because on slitlamp examination retraction of the posterior vitreous membrane was still lacking.

Photocoagulation: treatment is strongly advised. The arguments are the same as in the case of fig. 17. An extensive photocoagulation of all neovascularization foci and intraretinal haemorrhages was carried out (about $300 \times$, spot 3°).

Fig. 18b

The same area as on fig. 18a, 3 years after treatment. The fan of newly-formed vessels has almost disappeared.

Fig. 18c

Half a year later. At the upper border of the atrophic scar descrete loops of newly formed vessels are seen (arrows 1). Vitreous retraction, detectable by slitlamp examination, is causing a small preretinal haemorrhage (arrows 2).

Comment: one year after the first treatment a second treatment was necessary to destroy new small foci of neovascularization. The source of the haemorrhage seen on fig. 18c had to be coagulated twice before bleeding stopped definitely. In a follow-up period of six years no other complications did occur. Visual acuity deteriorated during this period from 1.0 to 0.5. The posterior pole never showed conspicuous changes. Ophthalmoscopically only a discrete depigmentation was seen. In the late phase of fluorography (3 min. after i.v. injection of the dye) a flower-shaped pattern of microcystic perimacular degeneration of the retina could be found. For the evolution of diabetic retinopathy in the left eye see fig. 27ab.

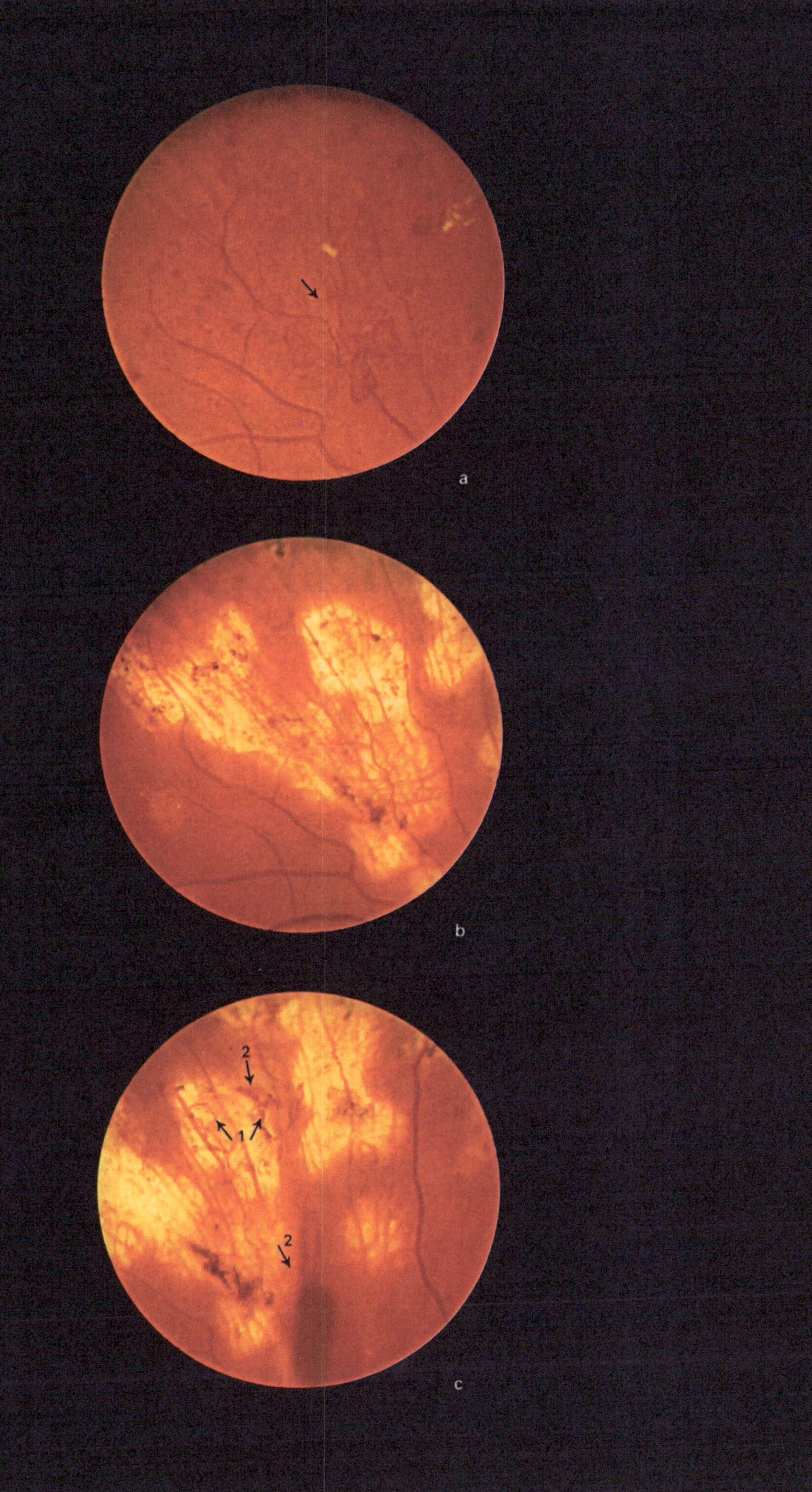

18

Fig. 19a (stereophotograph): N_2

Man, 22 years old, diabetes for 12 years. Left eye:
The big fan of newly-formed vessels on the nasal side of the disc is located preretinally.
This location is perceptable when fig. 19 is viewed in a stereoscopic way.
Visual acuity: 0.2.

Stage III, very advanced diabetic retinopathy with widespread and marked
neovascularization.

Prognosis: poor. The process of retraction of the posterior vitreous membrane
has already begun. Massive preretinal and vitreous haemorrhages are expected to
develop in due course. Moreover the diabetic arteriolopathy is very marked in this
case (see also the posterior pole of the same eye, fig. 14).

Photocoagulation: treatment is strongly advised. The arguments are the same
as for the treatment of the eyes presented on fig. 17ac and 18. In this case three
photocoagulations have been carried out: 1) $154 \times$, spot 4.5°; 2) one year later
$50 \times$, spot 4.5° and 3) $1\frac{1}{2}$ year after the first $60 \times$, spot 4.5°.

Fig. 19b (stereophotograph).
The same area as on fig. 19a 3 years after the first treatment. The vascular fan
has vanished. At the same site large atrophic coagulation-scars are seen and fibrous
strands in which some vessels can still be distinguished. The fibrous strands are
drawn forward by the retracting posterior membrane of the vitreous body. Their
preretinal location is easily seen when fig. 19b is viewed in a stereoscopic way.

Comment: In the observation period of 3 years after the first treatment no serious
complications occurred. Two additional sessions of treatment were necessary to
stabilize this very advanced and very progressive retinopathy. Visual acuity, already
poor at the beginning of the follow-up period (0.2), remained about the same:
0.15. Macular function was damaged by severe disturbance of the circulation at
the posterior pole (see fig. 14). For evolution of diabetic retinopathy in the right
eye see fig. 25.

19

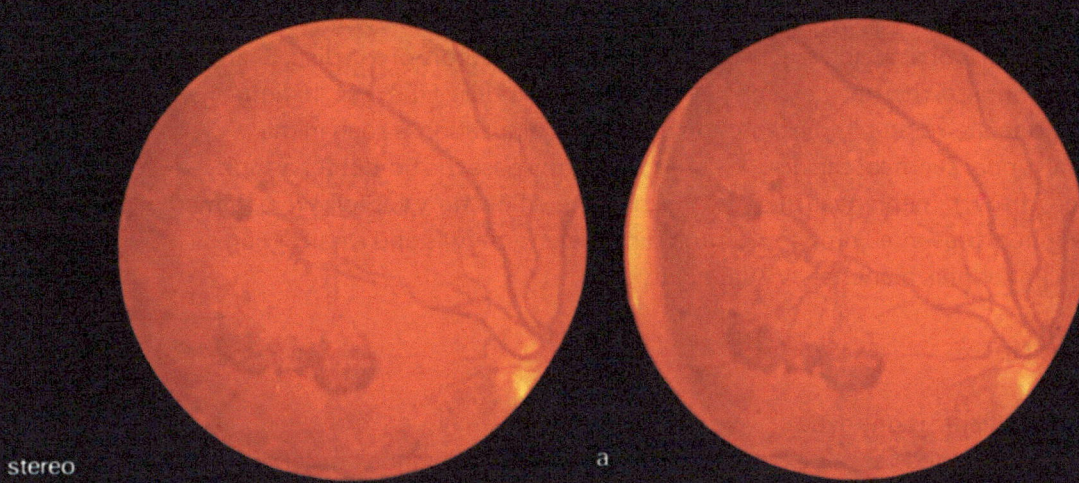

stereo   a

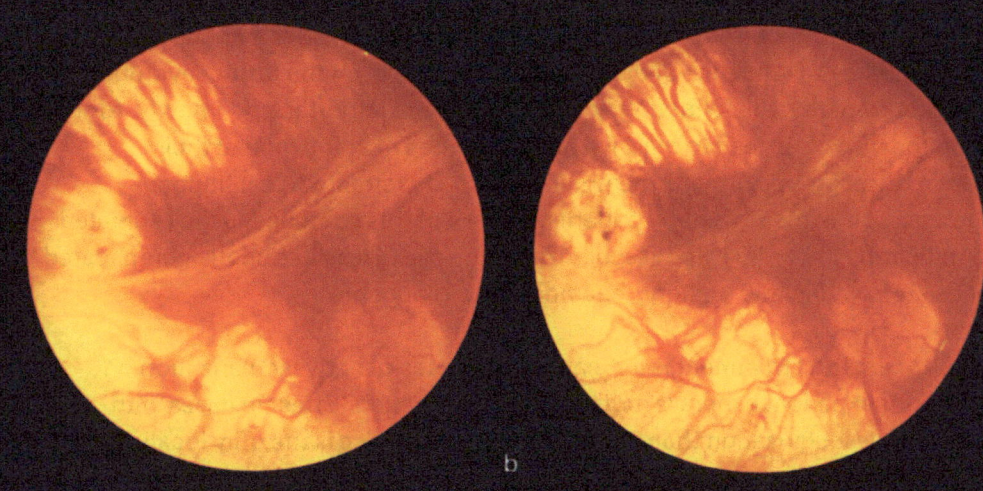

stereo   b

6 Neovascularization of the disc (Npap)

Fig. 20a: Npap₁

Man, 49 years old, diabetes for 19 years. Left eye:
The newly-formed vessels on the disc present themselves as a network or a sprout
of small vessel loops, which are located in one or more sectors of the disc. Even
in this early phase, they may extend just outside the border of the disc. In figure
20 this moderate (grade 1) presentation of neovascularization is seen in the
temporal-upper sector of the disc, where some loops pass the border for a short
distance (arrow). In this case this was the only site where new vessels were formed.
The periphery presented only some intraretinal haemorrhages and a narrowing of
the small arteriolar branches. Visual acuity: 1.0.

Fig. 21a: Npap₂

The same patient. Right eye:
When newly-formed vessels extend for a greater distance from the border of the
disc and their calibre becomes larger we speak about marked (grade 2)
neovascularization on the disc. Frequently at the same time vitreous retraction sets
in causing the first small haemorrhages (arrows).

Stage II, advanced diabetic retinopathy when moderate neovascularization on the
disc is present.

Stage III, very advanced diabetic retinopathy when marked neovascularization on
the disc is seen.

Prognosis: serious in cases with Npap₁ and worse in cases with Npap₂. When
we are to evaluate the influence of disc neovascularization on the further evolution
of diabetic retinopathy, the following considerations are important: (1) newly-formed
vessels on the disc often lead to massive haemorrhages. If at the time of their
appearance the posterior vitreous membrane is already retracted, as it happens
to be the case sometimes in elderly patients, the risk of this complication is estimated
to be significantly lower. (2) Neovascularization on the disc is frequently complicated
by rubeosis of the iris and ensuing haemorrhagic glaucoma.

Photocoagulation: treatment is indicated in all cases of neovascularization on
the disc. In our experience there is more chance of beneficial effect in cases with
multifocal neovascularization than in cases in which the disc is the only localization.
When neovascularization is localized on the disc only we coagulate in a straddling
way along the retinal veins. In the case of fig. 21a this technique has been applied
(181×, 4.5°).

Fig. 21b

The same eye as on fig. 21a 4 months after treatment. A conspicuous improvement
is seen: the haemorrhages have disappeared, the two neovascularization fans have
shrunk and fibrotic strands have developed (arrow).

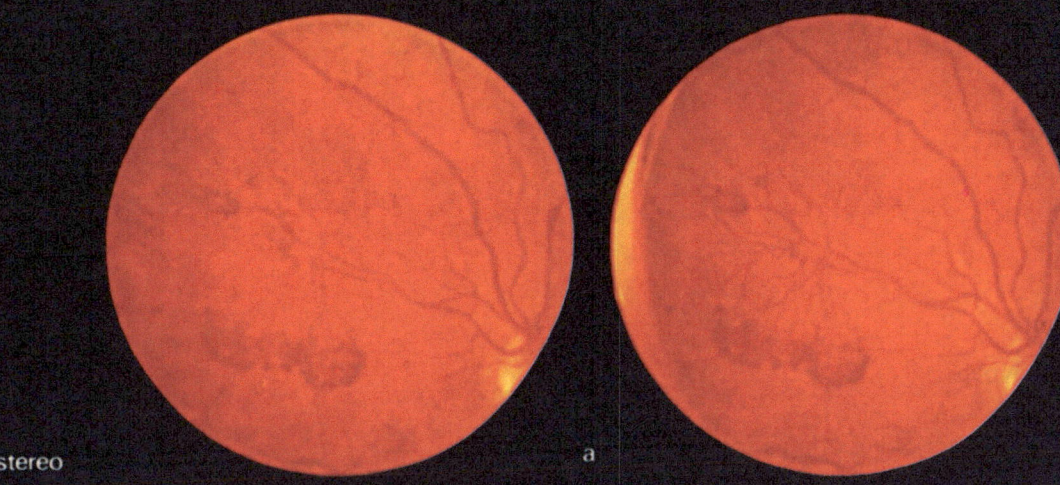

stereo   a

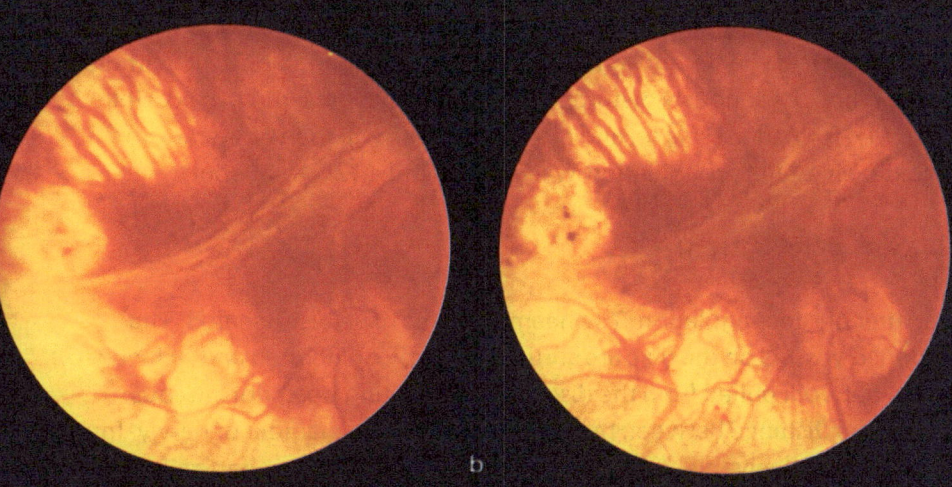

stereo   b

Fig. 20b

The same eye as on fig. 20a. This eye was not treated. Half a year later the neovascularization extended around the disc (arrows).

Comment: in the follow-up period of $1\frac{1}{2}$ year regression of neovascularization has been noticed in the treated, while progression was seen in the untreated eye. Visual acuity however deteriorated more in the treated right eye than in the untreated left eye. OD from 1.0 to 0.6; OS from 1.0 to 0.9.

Fig. 22a: Npap$_2$

Woman, 26 years old, diabetes for 16 years. Right eye:
The disc is surrounded by newly-formed vessels and a number of preretinal haemorrhages. Neovascularization, small preretinal and numerous intraretinal haemorrhages are spread over the whole of the posterior half of the retina, reaching their greatest density around the posterior pole. The veins are dilated, the small arterioles are narrowed. Visual acuity: 0.6.

Stage III, very advanced diabetic retinopathy with neovascularization.

Prognosis: serious. If neovascularization and preretinal haemorrhages continue, blindness is likely to occur.

Photocoagulation: treatment is strongly advised. By coagulating the pathologic areas of the retina the seriously disturbed circulation may recover. It is possible that the newly-formed vessels on and around the disc will then obliterate. In this case an extensive photocoagulation was carried out (320×, 3° spot).

Fig. 22b (stereophotograph)

One year after photocoagulation. The haemorrhages have disappeared. The newly-formed vessels on the disc are shrunken, partly obliterated and reduced to a yellowish network pulled from the disc by the retracting posterior vitreous membrane. The distance between the disc and this fine remainder of newly-formed vessels is easily perceivable when this figure is viewed stereoscopically.

Comment: the patient has been controlled for three years after treatment. The right eye remained quiet. No further photocoagulation was necessary. Three years after treatment the remainder of prepapillary neovascularization as seen on fig. 22b, could no longer be detected. The left eye which was not treated because the retinopathy was less marked, improved spontaneously. This happened to be one of our few cases in which spontaneous recovery of an advanced diabetic retinopathy with neovascularization could be observed. Visual acuity OD: 1.0; OS: 1.0.

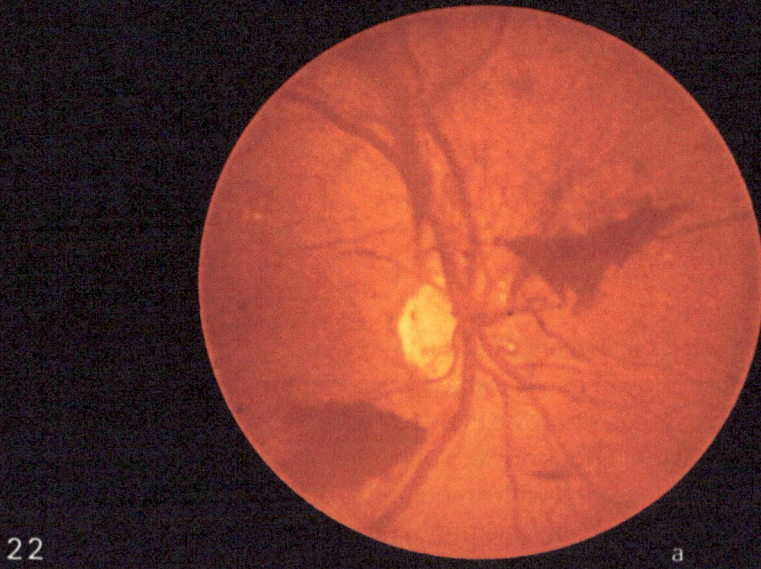

22

a

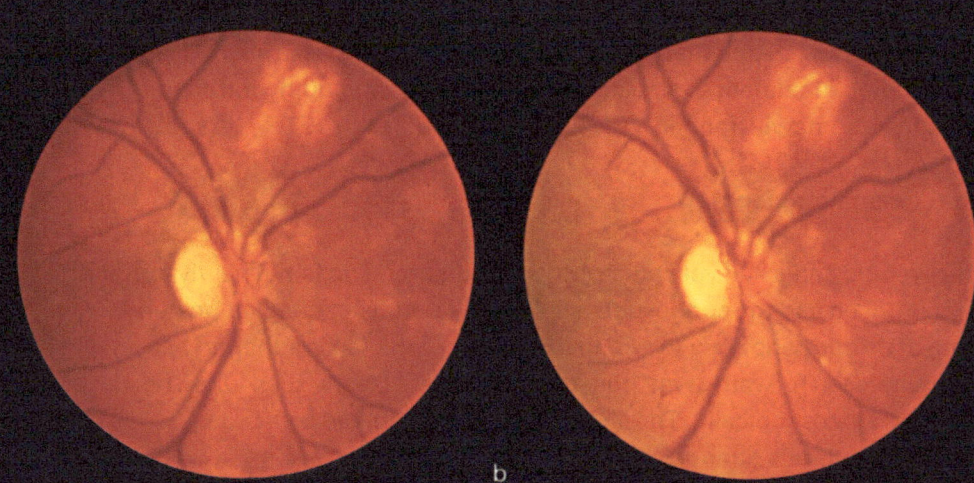

stereo

b

Fig. 23a: Npap > 2

Woman, 29 years old, diabetes for 9 years. Right eye:
A very large and very congested fan of newly formed vessels around the nasal
border of the disc. At the typical sites along the main temporal vessels but also
all around the mid-periphery of the fundus not less conspicuous neovascularization
is found. The veins are strongly engorged with irregularities of the vessel wall.
The arterioles are narrowed, the intraretinal haemorrhages extraordinarily numerous.
No hard exudates are seen. Fig. 23a presents the condition 2 months after treatment
with photocoagulation. Visual acuity: 0.3. Before treatment it was 0.8.

Stage III, very advanced diabetic retinopathy with extensive neovascularization.

Prognosis: poor. A favourable circumstance was the fact that photocoagulation
was performed at a moment at which vitreous retraction had not yet set in. On
account of this the newly-formed vessels could be coagulated efficiently.

Photocoagulation: treatment was strongly advised. In this case an almost complete
photocoagulation-treatment of all pathological changes, including intraretinal
haemorrhages and newly-formed vessels, was carried out (457 ×, 3° spot).

Fig. 23b (stereophotograph):

The same eye two and a half year after photocoagulation. The fan of newly-formed
vessels is shrunken and the congestion has disappeared. The retracted posterior
membrane of the vitreous body to which the border of the fan is adhering has
pulled the whole fan forward away from the disc. This is clearly seen when fig.
23b is viewed stereoscopically. The line of adhesion is marked by a broad
white-yellowish fibrous strand (arrows).

Comment: we had to deal in this case with an extremely progressive diabetic
retinopathy with very marked neovascularization. The posterior pole of the right
eye was however in a fairly good condition, as no tendency to obliteration of
the arterioles around the macula could be detected. Three years after the treatment
the condition of the right eye was regarded as quiet and stabilized. Visual acuity:
0.8. The visual acuity of the left eye of this patient was reduced to 1/300 at
the time of photocoagulation treatment of the right eye and remained unchanged
in the following three years.

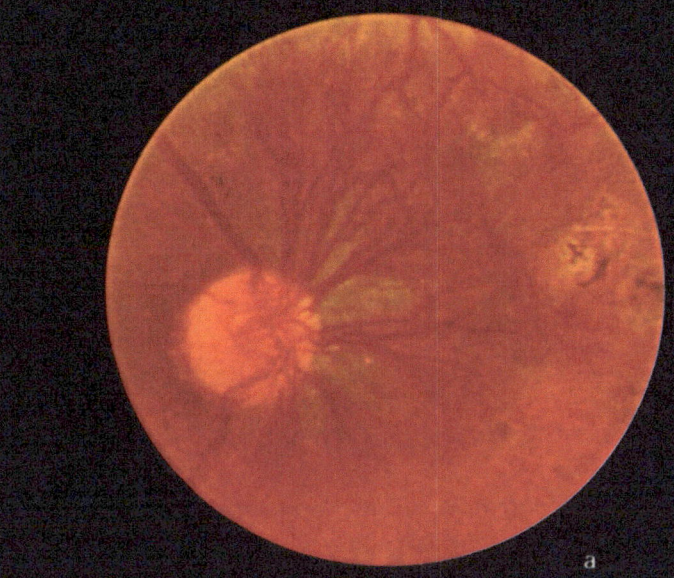

23

a

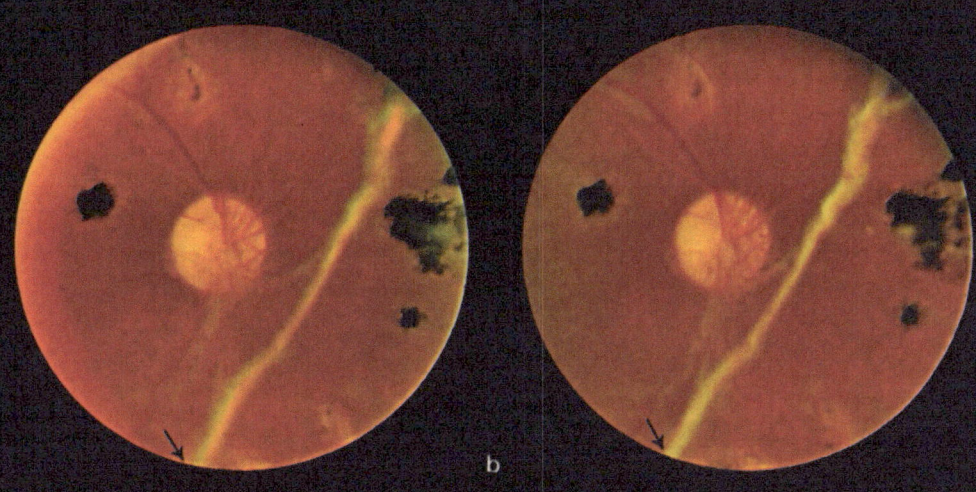

stereo

b

7 Proliferation of fibrous tissue (F)

Fig. 24: F_1

Woman, 25 years old, diabetes for 15 years. Left eye: avascular fibrous strands around the inferior part of the posterior pole. Arrows indicate the sites at which retinal vessels adhering to the strand are drawn forward.

Fig. 25: F_1 (stereophotograph)

Man, 22 years old, diabetes for 12 years. Right eye: early proliferation of fibrous tissue along newly-formed vessels next to the upper temporal vein.

Fibrous tissue mostly proliferates along newly-formed vessels which are pulled away from the surface of the retina by the retracting posterior vitreous membrane. The commencing or moderate fibrous proliferation (grade 1) is characterized by the appearance of gray-whitish strands around the posterior pole and near the optic disc. Ordinarily they have a sharp concave border which is touching the disc at its temporal or nasal side or which is passing over it. The concave border originates at the borderline between detached and still attached posterior vitreous surface. As the detachment of the posterior membrane of the vitreous body starts in the posterior part of the retina, the concave border in most cases surrounds the posterior pole as seen on fig. 24 and fig. 25. Its preretinal position, due to vitreous retraction is clearly seen on fig. 25 when viewed stereoscopically. In some cases the concave border is located on the nasal side of the disc.

Stage III, very advanced diabetic retinopathy.

Prognosis: in most of the cases prognosis is poor. Complications such as preretinal haemorrhages, retinoschisis and retinal detachment often occur. However, if fibrous proliferation is developing in a relatively quiet retina (as in fig. 24) complications may stay away for many years.

Photocoagulation: treatment is indicated when a progressive retinopathy is present. It should be extensive. The result is uncertain.

Comment: in the first case (fig. 24) retinopathy did not progress for as long as ten years. After this long quiet period neovascularization started again and small preretinal haemorrhages occurred. After photocoagulation treatment the eye was again stabilized. Visual acuity remained unchanged: 0.3. The other eye became blind through a haemorrhagic glaucoma.
In the second case (fig. 25) extensive photocoagulation was carried out at once. After recurrent preretinal haemorrhages and intrascleral diathermy a stabilization could be achieved with a visual acuity of 3/60. See fig. 14 and 19ab for the evolution of the left eye.

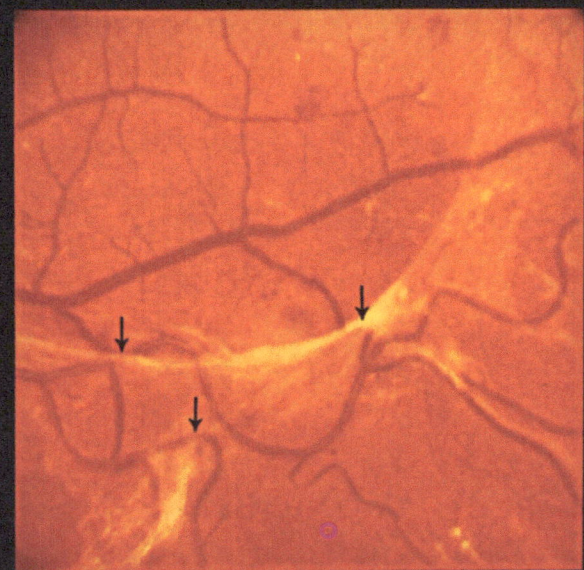

24

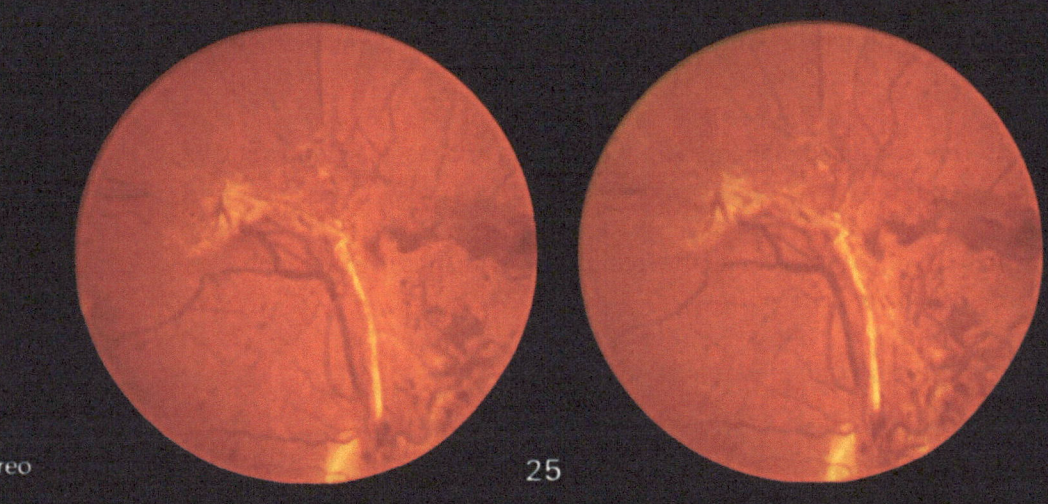

stereo   25

Fig. 26a: F₁

Woman, 50 years old, diabetes for 20 years. Left eye:

Just perceivable fibrous strand at the level of the retina along the upper temporal vessels (arrows). Neovascularization and preretinal haemorrhages above the disc. The veins are engorged and tortuous, a collateral vein is emerging along the upper temporal vein. Visual acuity: 0.5.

Stage III, very advanced diabetic retinopathy with neovascularization and early fibrosis.

Prognosis: poor. Progression of the retinopathy with massive preretinal haemorrhages is very likely.

Photocoagulation: treatment is strongly advised.

Fig. 26b

One year after photocoagulation. Next to the pigmented coagulation scars a membrane formed of fibrous or glial tissue is seen (arrows).

Comment: the left eye of the patient remained quiet for six years after treatment. Visual acuity: 0.4. The right eye at the time of treatment showed a more advanced stage of evolution with very marked fibrous proliferation. Despite photocoagulation a partial retinal detachment developed. The visual acuity 6 years after treatment was 1/60.

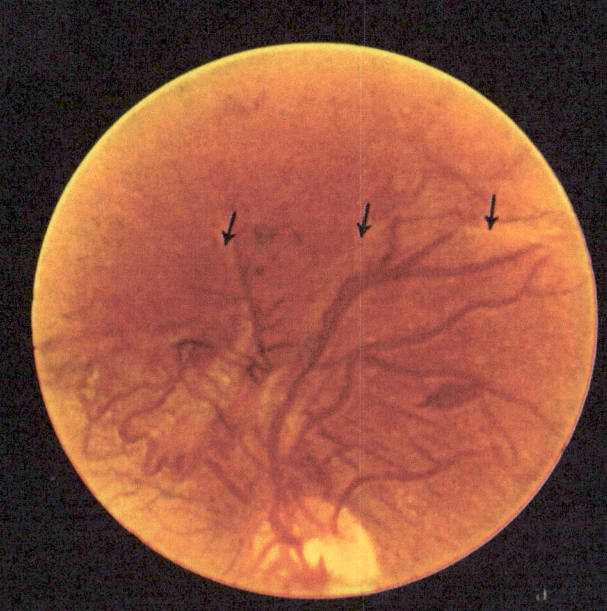

26

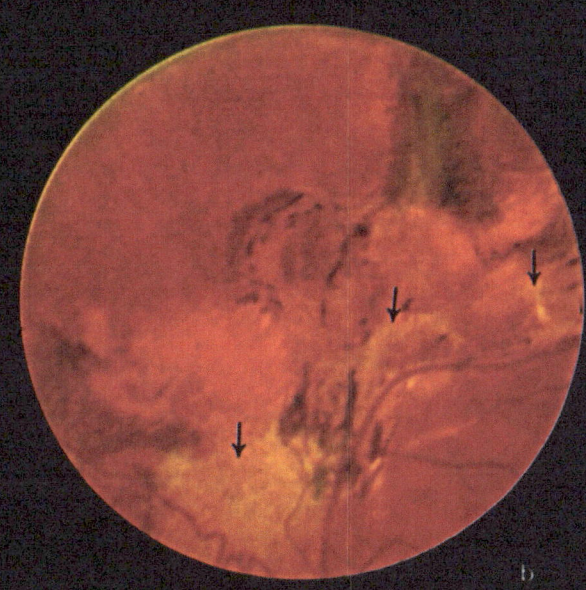

42

Fig. 27ab: F₂

Man, 26 years old, diabetes for 24 years. Left eye:
A tongslike fibrous proliferation is seen around the posterior pole. The time lapse
between the two photographs is one year. Visual acuity: 0.1. The late phase of
fibrous proliferation (F₂) is characterized by shrinkage of the fibrous strands and
increasing retraction of the posterior vitreous membrane. The consequence of this
shrinking process is clearly seen when we compare the diameter and the shape
of the fibrous ring on photographs 27a and b.

Stage IV, final stage of diabetic retinopathy.

Prognosis: in most cases poor, but in a few cases reasonably good. If retraction
of the vitreous and massive haemorrhages do not occur, a stabilization may be
reached with a still useful visual acuity.

Photocoagulation: treatment is indicated if it seems possible to destroy the
newly-formed vessels. This may prevent massive preretinal haemorrhages and hold
back further progression of the retinopathy. In this case an extensive photocoagulation
was carried out.

Comment: the eye remained quiet until the time of publication — six years after
treatment. Visual acuity did not deteriorate further: 0.1.

Fig. 28: (stereophtoograph): F₂

Man, 54 years old, diabetes for 13 years. Left eye:
The retracting posterior vitreous membrane is pulling a branch of the temporo-superior
vein and a neovascular sail above the optic disc. The temporo-superior vein and
the superficial layer of the adjacent retina are also retracted from the normal level
of the fundus. This is clearly seen when the figure is viewed stereoscopically.
Visual acuity: 1/60.

Stage IV, final stage of the diabetic retinopathy with retinal detachment.

Prognosis: hopeless. Blindness is caused by massive haemorrhages as in this
case or by retinal detachment.

Photocoagulation: treatment is useless.

Comment: the eye became completely blind due to a massive vitreous haemorrhage,
shortly after this photograph was taken.

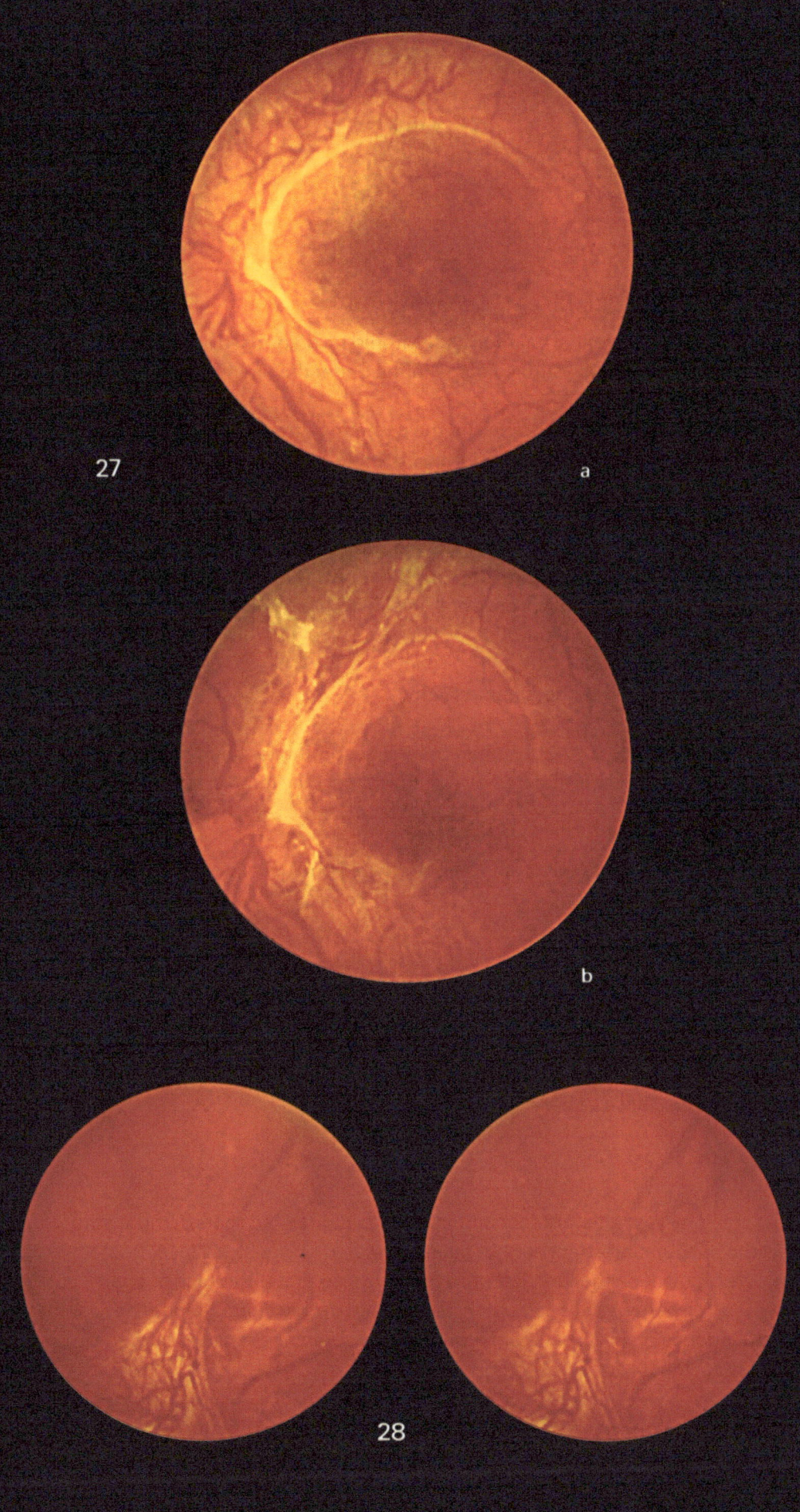

27   a

b

stereo   28

8 Preretinal haemorrhages (H)

Fig. 29a: H_1

Man, 34 years old, diabetes for 14 years. Left eye:
A moderate (grade 1) preretinal haemorrhage should be diagnosed when a
haemorrhage is located on the surface of the retina under the internal limiting

membrane, or between this membrane and the posterior vitreous membrane. The
same gradation is used when the haemorrhage is small and does not diffuse into
the vitreous body, or is only partly diffusing so that the fundus can still be examined.
When the space between retina and posterior vitreous membrane is narrow the
blood forms a sharply circumscribed blot as seen on fig. 29a. (Notice the slight
prominence when viewed stereoscopically.) When there is more space the bloodfilled
pocket is sickle-shaped or takes a horizontal level with the typical 'Napoleon's
hat'-configuration as seen on fig. 30a.

Stage III, very advanced diabetic retinopathy.

Prognosis: serious. There may be however a fair absorbing tendency. Visual acuity
may remain unchanged, or, if affected by haemorrhage, may recover within a relative
short time.

Photocoagulation: treatment is definitely indicated and usually exerts a favourable
influence on further evolution.

Fig. 29b (stereophotograph):

The haemorrhage of fig. 29a one day after photocoagulation. The coagulations
seem to lie superficially in the blood layer when viewed stereoscopically. Notice
the position of the coagulations in relation to the underlying vessels. An attempt
was made to spare these vessels.

Fig. 29c

The same area one year after photocoagulation. The pigmented scars demonstrate
now that the coagulating effect has not been hampered by the blood layer from
reaching the pigment epithelium. One may observe also that the course of one
of the vessels (arrow) was not accurately recognized during coagulation. The present
scar gives evidence of this. But no unfavourable consequences ensued from this
coagulation accident.

Comment: in the follow-up period of two and a half years no preretinal
haemorrhages occurred. However some more coagulating sessions with the Argon
laser were necessary to destroy new neovascularization foci. Visual acuity of both
eyes remained 1.0.

29

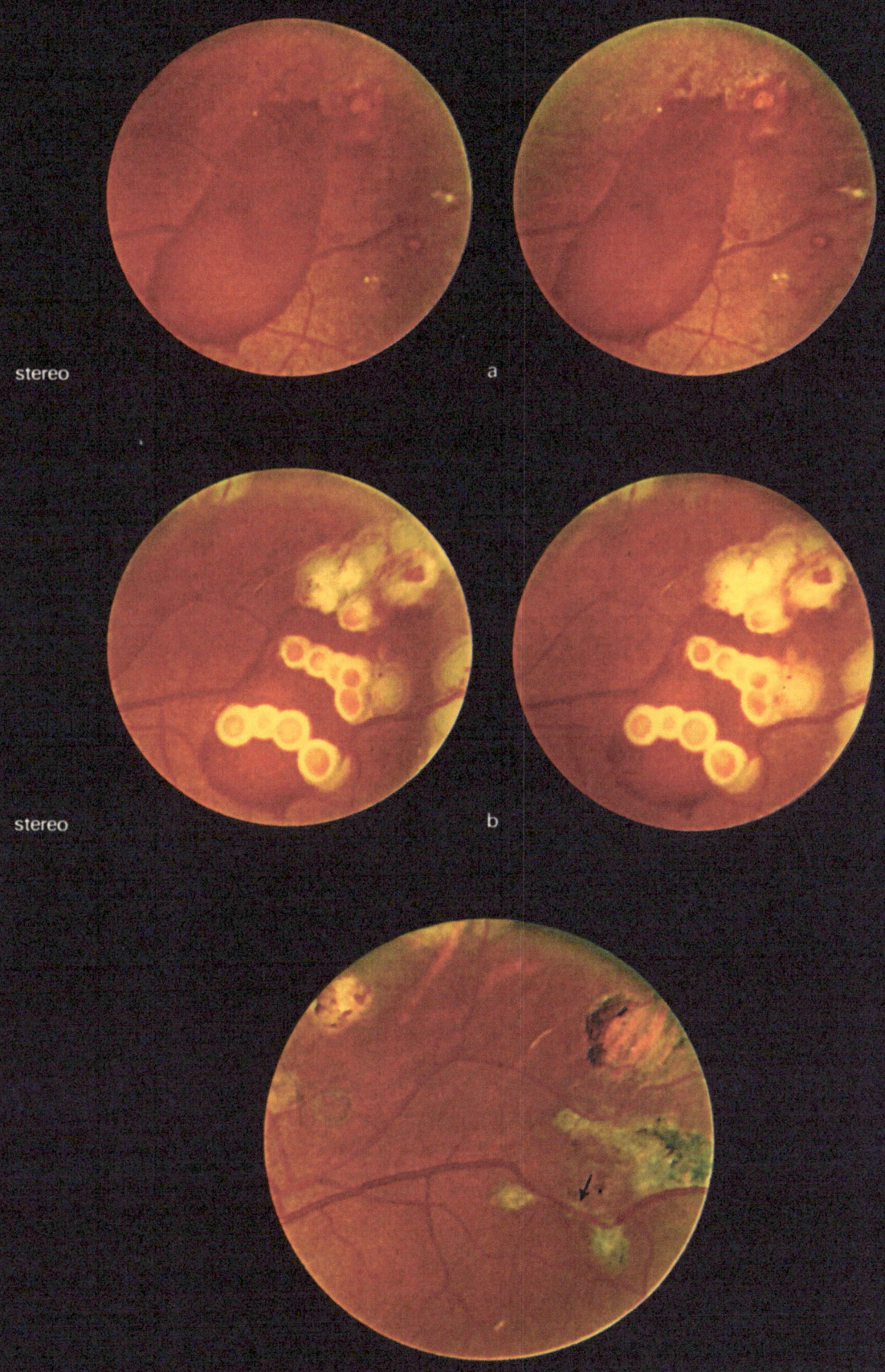

stereo

a

stereo

b

c

Fig. 30a: H₁

Woman, 42 years old, diabetes for 12 years. Left eye:
A preretinal haemorrhage with horizontal level is seen temporally to the macular
area. The commencing detachment of the vitreous at the posterior pole has provided
just enough space for the blood to settle and to form a horizontal level. No lesion
of the macular area is seen. Visual acuity: 1.0.

Stage III, very advanced diabetic retinopathy.

Prognosis: serious. There may be however a fair absorbing tendency. Visual acuity
may remain unchanged, or, if affected by haemorrhage, may recover within a relative
short time.

Photocoagulation: treatment is strongly advised. In most cases it is possible
to exert a favourable influence on further evolution. In this case an extensive treatment
was carried out.

Fig. 30b

One day after photocoagulation. The haemorrhage has changed its shape. A part
seems already absorbed. It is obvious that some of the newly-formed vessels have
been left untreated.

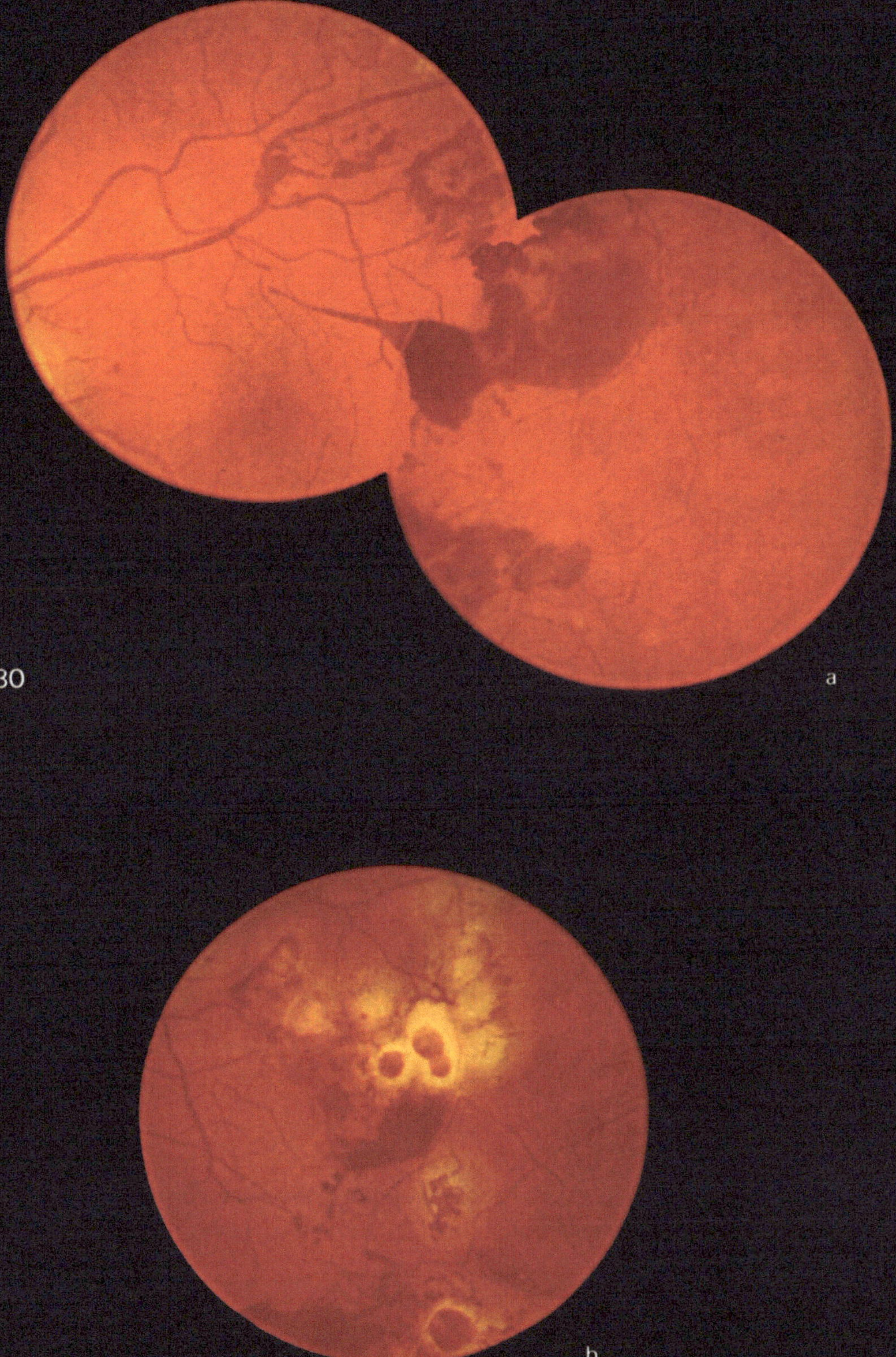

30

a

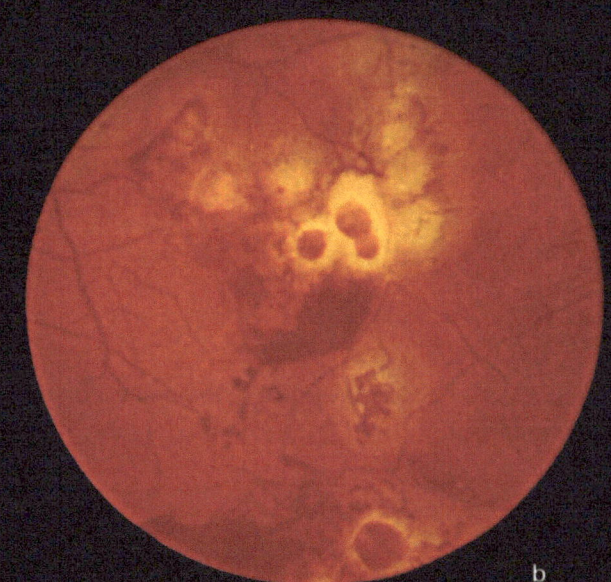

b

Fig. 30c

One year after photocoagulation. The arrows point to the enlarged network of newly-formed vessels, spared during the first photocoagulating session.

Fig. 30d

After an additional treatment the network of newly-formed vessels disappeared (arrow).

Comment: in this case three photocoagulation sessions in both eyes have been carried out. The progression of the diabetic retinopathy was controlled during the follow-up period of three years. No serious complications occurred. Visual acuity of both eyes however, deteriorated slowly to 0.6. This was due to the enlargement of the areas of capillary closure around the macula.

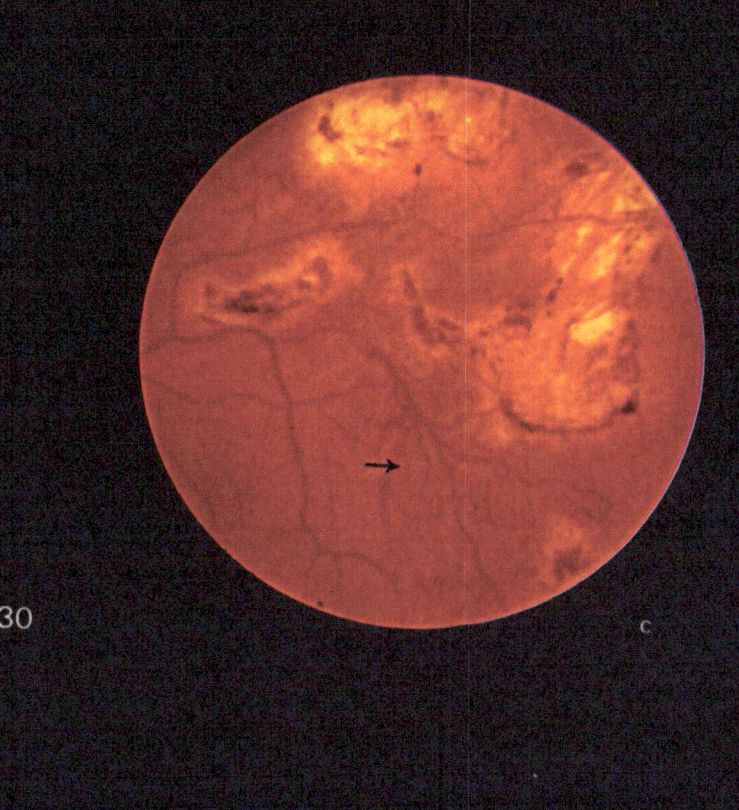

30

c

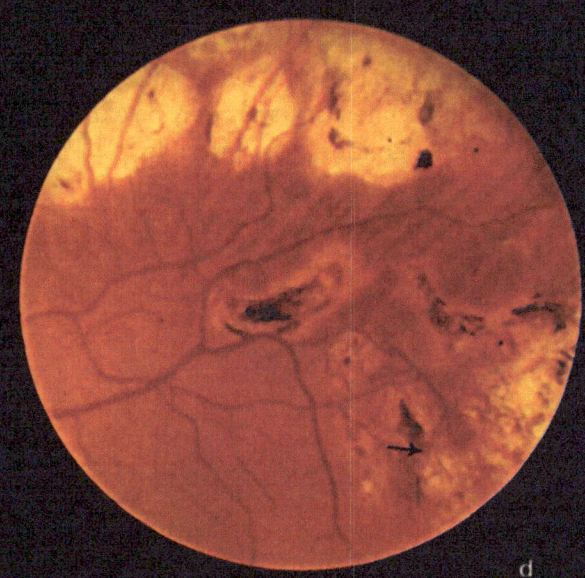

d

Fig. 31a: H$_2$

Woman, 29 years old, diabetes for 13 years. Right eye:
A very marked, grade 2, preretinal haemorrhage should be diagnosed, when a
preretinal haemorrhage is abundant and diffusion of blood cells into the vitreous
body occurs to such an extent that part of the fundus is clouded. If the haemorrhage
is so abundant that the fundus is totally clouded and details can no longer be
observed, we speak of a massive, grade >2, vitreous haemorrhage.

Stage III, very advanced diabetic retinopathy with neovascularization and
commencing retraction of the posterior vitreous membrane.

Prognosis: poor. Absorption of the blood cells and clearing up of the vitreous
body occurs only very slowly. Recurrent haemorrhages may be expected; if they
are frequent and abundant, resorption is not longer possible.

Photocoagulation: treatment is strongly advised as soon as the source or sources
of haemorrhage can be detected. If applied at the right moment, photocoagulation
can be really beneficial by preventing further haemorrhages. If applied after repeated
haemorrhages happened, the benefit of treatment becomes questionable. In this
case photocoagulation was carried out at once. Besides the source of the haemorrhage
on the nasal border of the disc (see arrow in fig. 31 b and c) all pathologic areas
in the fundus were treated.

Fig. 31d

One year after treatment. Fibrous strands above and below the disc are the only
remainders of the peripapillary neovascularization and the abundant haemorrhage.

Comment: during the follow-up time of five years additional treatment of this
eye was not necessary. The left eye had to be treated 3 times at intervals of
several months. After this the retina remained quiet during a follow-up period of
four years. Visual acuity OD: 0.3; OS: 1.0.

31

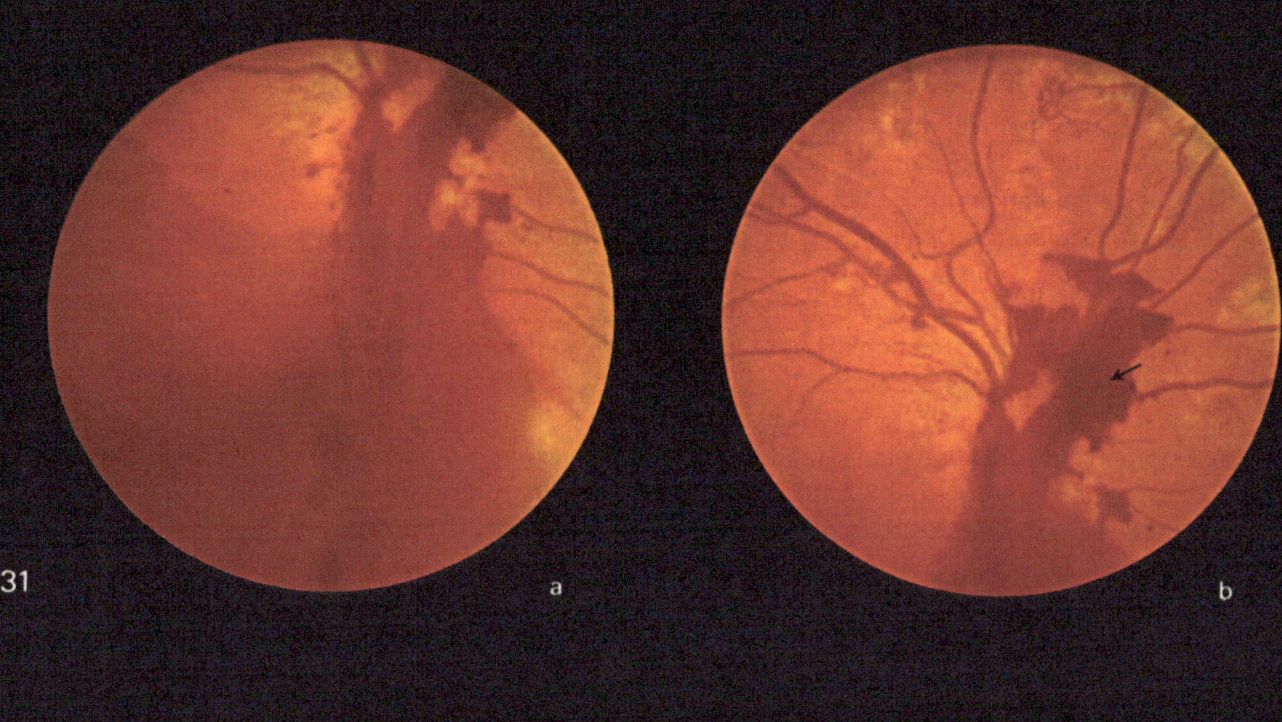

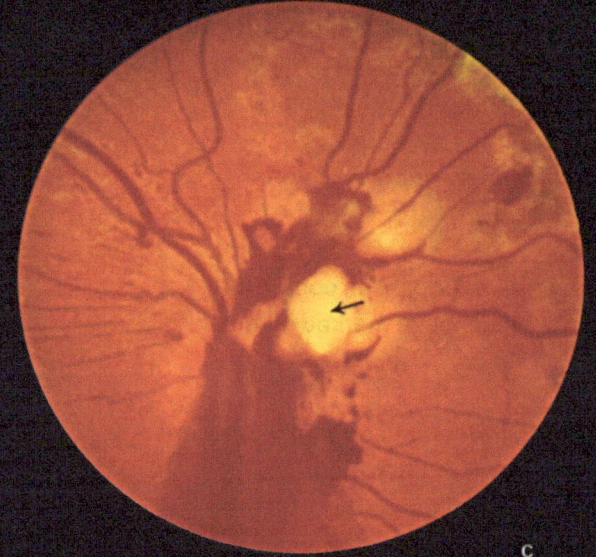

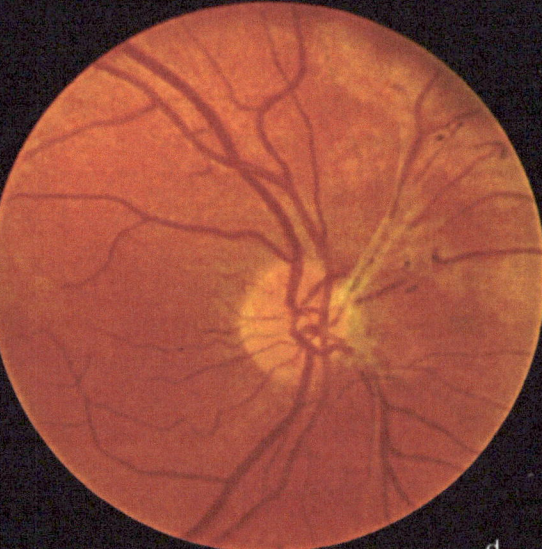

9 Lesions of the macular area

In the course of a diabetic retinopathy the macular area may be affected by different pathological changes:
1 Haemorrhages: intraretinal, preretinal, subretinal, varying in size and number.
2 Exudates: small and numerous, or large, solitary and discoid.
3 Oedema: diffuse, cystic or schisislike.
4 'Dry' degeneration: this condition is characterized by discrete pigment dislocation in the macular area. On fluorography, areas of capillary closure and in the late phase (about 3 minutes after dye injection) a flower-shaped pattern of microcystic lesions may be found around the macula.
5 Retina folds: due to traction of fibrous proliferation on the surface of the retina temporal to the macular area.

As morphologic differentiation in moderate (grade 1) and marked (grade 2) presentation of these lesions is difficult, we prefer to evaluate the macular condition on the basis of the corrected visual acuity if at least no other cause for visual disturbance is present (for instance, cataract or vitreal opacities).
If visual acuity is between 0.8 and 0.5, a moderate, or grade 1 macular lesion is diagnosed. If visual acuity ranges from 0.4 to 5/60 we speak of a marked, or grade 2 macular lesion. If visual acuity is less than 5/60 we speak of a very marked, or more than grade 2 macular lesion.
The limit between the marked and moderate macular lesions have been arbitrarily put at a visual acuity of 0.5. We have chosen 0.5 because with a visual acuity of less than 0.5 reading and writing become difficult. For some of our patients beyond this limit 'economic' blindness sets in.

On the basis of the macular lesions we classify the clinical picture as:
Stage III, advanced diabetic retinopathy, when a moderate, grade 1, lesion of the macula is present (visual acuity: 0.8–0.5),
Stage III, very advanced diabetic retinopathy, when a marked, grade 2, lesion of the macula is present (visual acuity: 0.4–5/60).

Prognosis: in the presence of moderate macular lesions – serious. The condition may however remain unchanged for many years. In the presence of marked macular lesions – poor. Further deterioration is most likely to occur.

Photocoagulation: treatment is in general indicated in moderate and marked lesions of the macular area. It may be beneficial by reducing oedema, exudates and intraretinal haemorrhages. Photocoagulation has a kind of 'draining effect' on the retina at the posterior pole which may improve its function.
The Argon laser, combined with slitlamp observation, provides at present the most appropriate technical device to treat the perifoveal area.
When lesions in the macula are so marked that visual acuity is less than 5/60, photocoagulation can hardly be expected to improve macular function. It may however be necessary to treat other areas of the fundus with neovascularization in order to prevent an evolution towards massive haemorrhages and complete blindness.

Table with classification examples of diabetic retinopathy

Ex.Nr.	ma+h	e	mac	A	V	N	Npap	F	H	CV	Rub	Stage	Progn.	Therapy
1	0–1	1	0	0	0	0	0	0	0	0	0	I	good	—
2	1–2	1	0	0	1	0	0	0	0	0	0	II	doubtful	LC
3	2	2	2	1	1	0	0	0	0	0	0	III	serious	LC+laser
4	2	0	0	1	1	1	0	0	0	0	0	II+neov.	serious	LC
5	2	2	2	1	1–2	1	0	0	0	0	0	III+neov.	poor	LC+laser
6	2	0	0	1	2	2	0	0	1	1	0	III+neov.	poor	LC
7	2	2	2	1	1	1	0	0	0	0	0	III+neov.	poor	LC+laser
8	1	1	0	2	1	0	2	1	1	1	1	III–IV	poor	LC
9	1	1	1	2	2	1	>2	1	1	1	2	IV	very poor	LC+laser
10	1	1	2	>2	>2	2	1	>2	2	2+	1	IV	hopeless	—

Abbreviations:

Ex.Nr.	example number
ma	microaneurysms
h	intraretinal haemorrhages
e	lipoid deposits or hard exudates
mac	condition of the macula
A	condition of arteries
V	condition of veins
N	neovascularization of the retina
Npap	neovascularization of the disc
F	proliferation of fibrous tissue
H	preretinal and vitreous haemorrhages
CV	retraction of vitreous body
Rub	rubeosis of the iris
Stage	developmental stage of diabetic retinopathy
Progn.	prognosis based upon natural course of the disease left without photocoagulation treatment
Therapy	indication to treatment
Lc	light coagulation

Some guide lines to photocoagulation treatment of diabetic retinopathy

Plan of treatment — general considerations

In order not to overlook pathological changes it is advisable to proceed following a fixed scheme. Figure 32 gives an outline of such a procedure, which in our experience has proved to be quite suitable. We start beneath the disc and treat sector by sector, in the sequence indicated by the numbers, finishing with the area around the posterior pole. In each sector we begin near the border of the disc and proceed along the vessels towards the periphery. Frequent control by indirect ophthalmoscopy is indispensable, especially when treating the area around the posterior pole.

The 3 degree light spot provides the most suitable diameter. Around the posterior pole a smaller spotdiameter should be used, not only to protect the function of the macula, but also to spare as much as possible the very fine meshwork of retinal vessels situated temporal to the macular area.

The number of coagulations carried out during one session of treatment may be as many as 400, without taking the risk of serious functional damage to the retina. It is also advisable to keep away from the macula at a distance of at least 1 to 1/2 disc diameter from its border. We are convinced that a complete cover of all pathological changes except those near the macula is essential for achieving a stabilization in a progressive retinopathy.

If we need for treatment of the nasal half of the fundus more than 200 coagulations it is advisable to postpone the treatment of the temporal half to a second session after some days.
If the treatment of the periphery has been very extensive the retina around the posterior pole should not be treated in the same session. It is better to supplement photocoagulation of the posterior pole several months later on the basis of the fluorographic findings. If available, the Argon laser is preferred.

A repetition of the coagulation treatment is often necessary. The interval between the first and the second session may vary between several months and several years. If the follow-up period is long enough, discrete signs of re-activity may appear in almost all of successfully treated and stabilized cases.

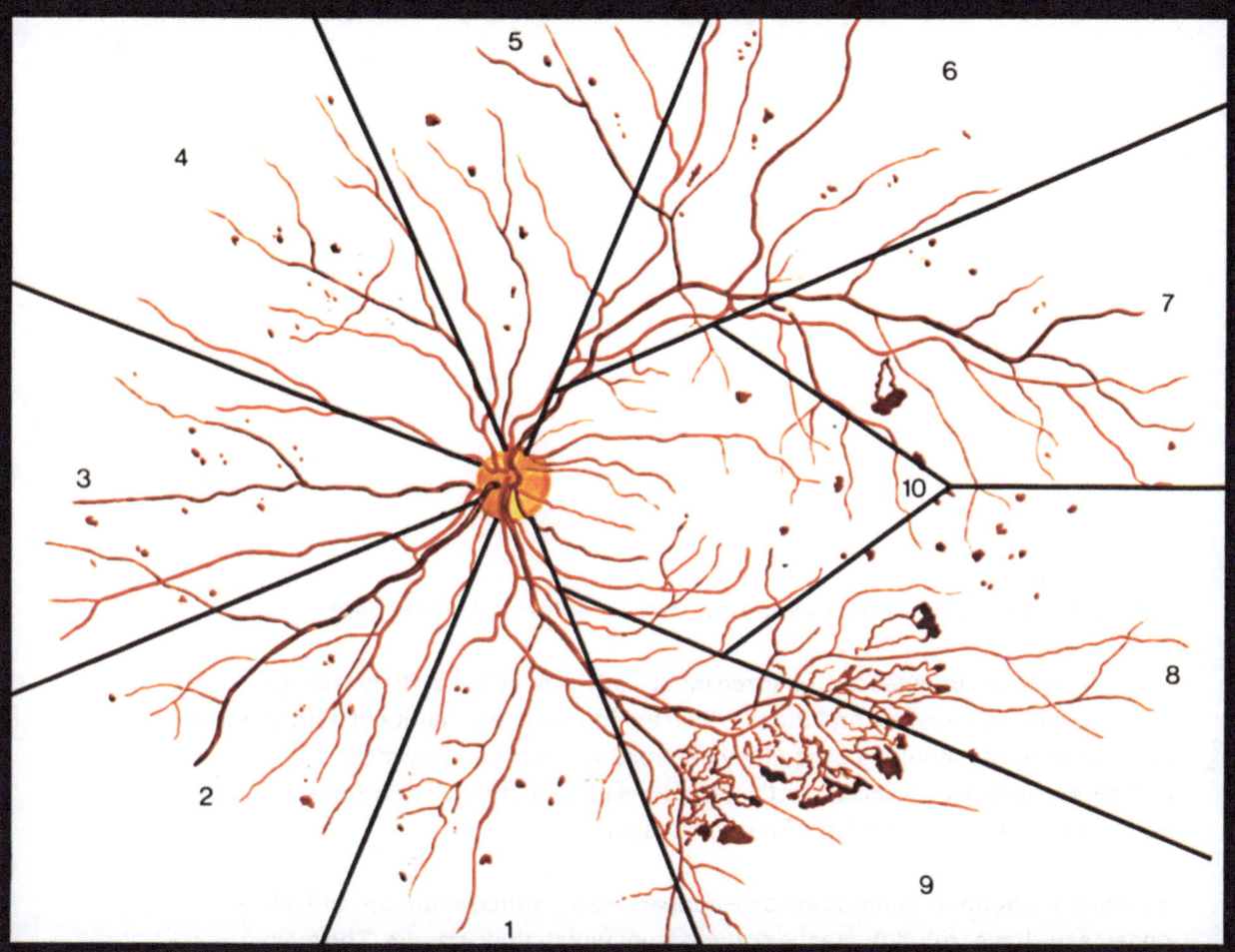

Treatment of intraretinal haemorrhages, microaneurysms and exudates

Intraretinal haemorrhages are localized most likely at sites of capillary leakage. Grouped microaneurysms and those which are found in the vicinity of hard exudates indicate areas of pathological capillary network. On fluorography most microaneurysms leak; consequently we may assume that they contribute to retinal oedema and to the formation of hard exudates.

To make intraretinal haemorrhages disappear and to reduce exudates and retinal oedema we have to coagulate the sources from which they emerge. The main targets for photocoagulation in non-proliferative diabetic retinopathy are therefore intraretinal haemorrhages and grouped microaneurysms (see figures 33 and 34).

The coagulation of hard exudates and cotton-wool spots is useless. On the border of old cotton-wool patches, however, very often a dilatation and proliferation of capillaries is observed. From this point of view it is advisable to coagulate around cotton-wool spots in order to prevent future neovascularization (see arrows in figures 33 and 34).

Treatment of neovascularization of the retina

Networks of newly-formed vessels have to be attacked directly. The whole area of the network should be coagulated sparing only the vessels which belong to the normal retinal vasculature (see fig. 35). When the neovascularization is widespread, and extensive coagulation seems necessary, we have to be aware that an exudative reaction of the choroid may occur and may lead to a partial detachment of the retina or to a detachment of the choroid. Though the detachment subsides mostly within a week we should avoid this complication by spreading the coagulations in such a way that small parts of the retina in between are spared.

33

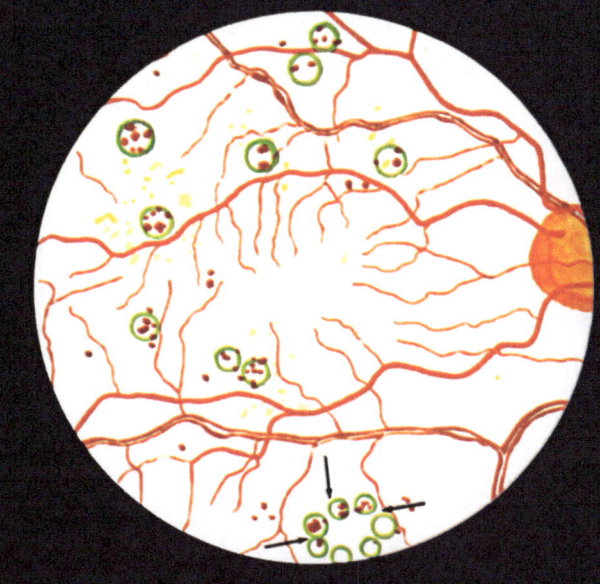

34

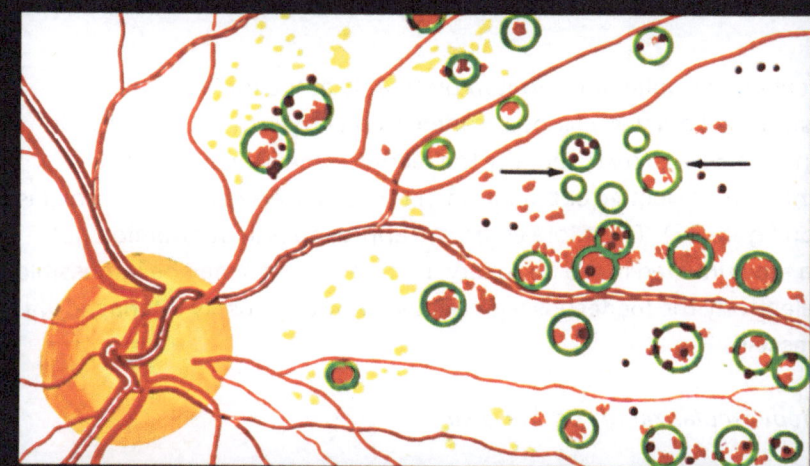

35

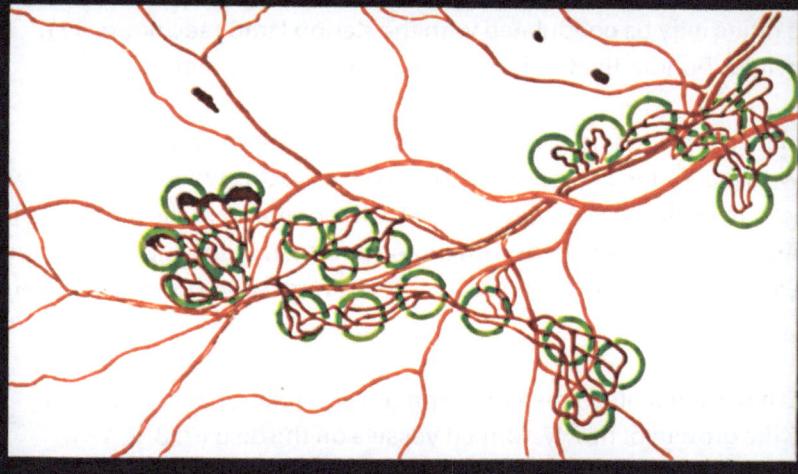

If we have to treat neovascular fans we start preferably at the top and finish at
the foot of the stretched out vessel loops as indicated with arrows 1 in figure 36.
In very large fans it is wise to try to identify the feeder vessels by means of
fluorography and apply selective coagulation of those vessels using the Argon laser
(see arrows 2 on figure 36). This more elaborate approach is in our opinion not
necessary if the fan is located in the periphery. In many cases it may be impossible
to coagulate selectively the feeder vessels because they are closely interlaced with
the collector vessels.

Treatment of neovascularization on the disc

Small newly-formed tufts or networks of vessels within the border of the disc
are not coagulated.

Fronds of newly-formed vessels passing the border of the disc and located in
the plane of the retina may be coagulated with the Xenon lamp (see figure 37).
However nerve fiber bundle field defects may be the consequence.

If the neovascularization encompasses the greater part of the border of the disc
a coagulation with the Xenon arc is not advisable because this would create very
large field defects. In such cases one should try to determine by means of fluorography
the feeder vessels and coagulate them with the Argon laser, following the method
advocated by Little, Zweng and l'Espérance (4, 5, 6). This technique may be seen
in figure 38.

Several authors have advocated ablative peripheral coagulation of the retina in
order to reduce the growth of newly-formed vessels on the disc (7, 8, 9, 18).
In our experience less extensive coagulation close along the retinal veins as shown
in figure 39, and also in the vicinity of the arterio-venous crossings, may have
a beneficial effect too on neovascularization arising from the disc (case of figure
26a, b).

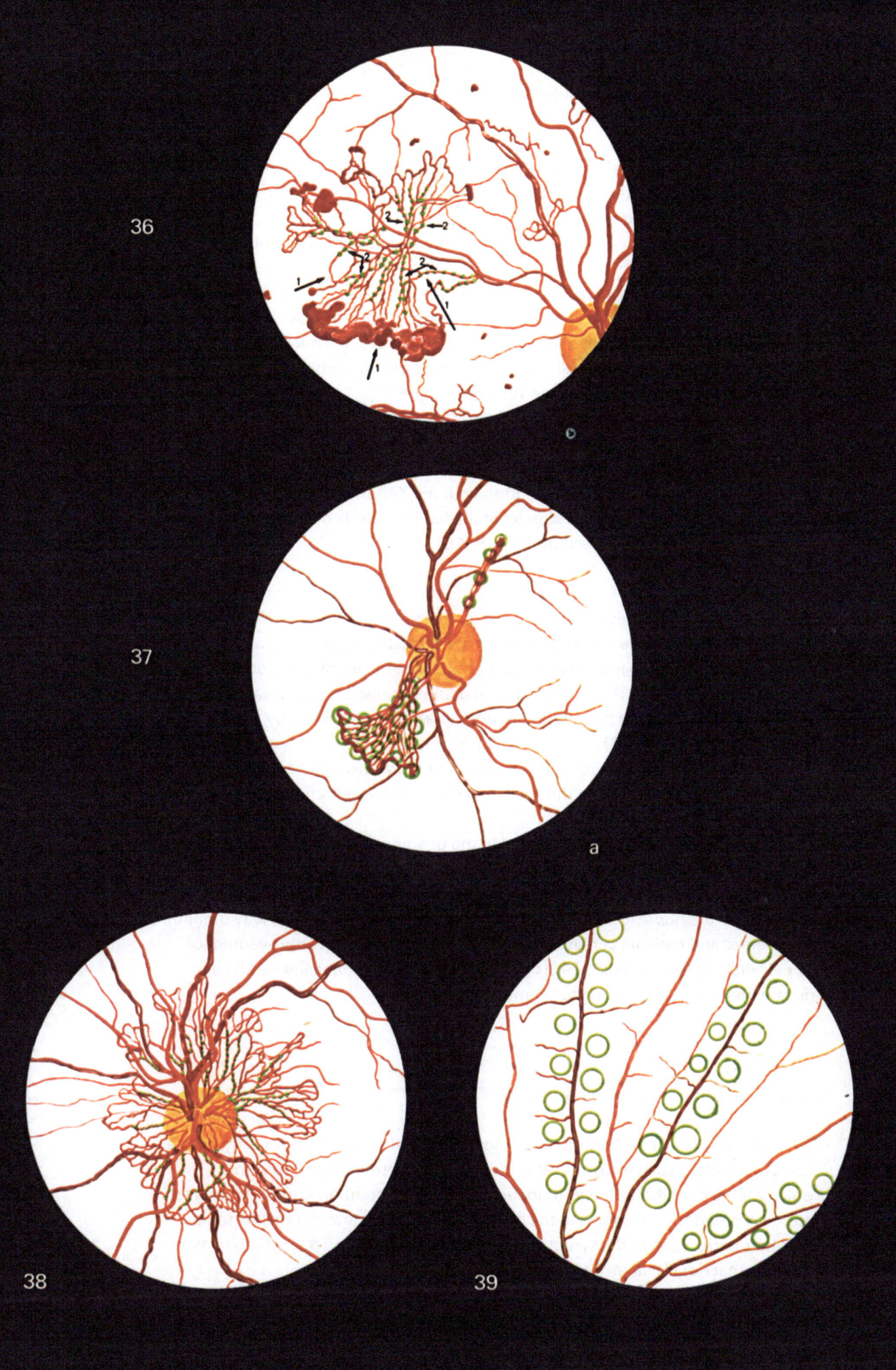

36

37

a

38

39

Some difficulties in photocoagulation treatment

a Preretinal haemorrhages
In order to treat a preretinal haemorrhage adequately we have to locate its source. This is not at all easy if the source is covered by blood or if it is at some distance from a sickle-shaped preretinal haemorrhage.
In the first case we may try to attack the source by coagulating the overlying blood layer.
In sickle-shaped haemorrhages a thin curved blood line which is connected with one of the ends of the sickle may indicate the site of the source.
As a general rule for treatment of preretinal haemorrhages one may state: if the source is visible the patient should be treated as soon as possible. Subsequent haemorrhages may hide the source for ever.

b Retracted newly-formed vessels
If newly-formed vessels are drawn away from the plane of the retina by the retracting posterior vitreous membrane, coagulation with the Xenon lamp may become impossible. In such cases the occlusion of the feeder vessels by the Argon laser has been proven to be successful (4, 5, 6, 10).

c Macular lesions
Before starting direct coagulation of the area around the macula we should remember that the circulation in the capillary network at the posterior pole may improve following a widespread treatment of the periphery of the fundus and occasionally also spontaneously (11, 12). Improvement of the fluorescein angiographic picture of the posterior pole after peripheral treatment has been described by Meyer-Schwickerath (13).
Therefore in cases of advanced retinopathy in which widespread coagulation of the whole fundus is necessary the central parts should be left untreated during the first session.
However, if the retinopathy is restricted to the posterior pole, a direct approach of the lesions is inevitable. The utmost accuracy in treating the leaking areas of the capillary network is achieved while using the Argon laser and referring during treatment to the fluorescein angiograms of the posterior pole. In this way diminution of exudates and oedema can be achieved. Sometimes even an improvement of visual acuity is encountered (14, 15, 16, 17). In our experience the results are poor when visual acuity is less than 5/60.

Discussion
Evaluation of symptoms and prognosis

The main purpose of evaluating the clinical picture of diabetic retinopathy on the basis of a code system is to draw attention to all symptoms separately. In a polymorphic condition such as diabetic retinophaty, attention is easily drawn to more conspicuous symptoms at the cost of less obvious ones. If one has to put numbers under each of the symptoms in the scheme given on page 22, one may feel sure that details have not been overlooked.
Details easily overlooked but important for prognosis are for instance the constriction of small arterial branches, the commencing of beading of the veins, the retraction

of the posterior vitreous membrane. A fixed scheme provides too a basis for comparing
the clinical data of different observers. This purpose is not less important than
the first one, as complete unanimity regarding the therapeutic approach to diabetic
retinopathy is not yet reached.

Evaluation of the clinical picture includes the prediction of its further evolution.
This is done on the basis of the prognostic value of the different symptoms and
their combinations:

a Microaneurysms and intraretinal haemorrhages

If microaneurysms and intraretinal haemorrhages are numerous, widespread and
accompanied by engorged veins and cotton-wool spots, progression of retinopathy
is very likely.
Neovascularization may develop in future (case of fig. 1, 2, 3). If, at the same
time, the small arterial branches are narrowed or occasionally occluded, a severe
deterioration of the retinal circulation and a marked neovascularization may be
expected in the near future (case of figure 4).

b Lipoid exudates

Numerous fatty exudates spread in a wide area around the disc and the posterior
pole and accompanied by intraretinal haemorrhages and engorged veins point to
a severe disturbance of the retinal circulation. Not only has progression of exudation
to be expected, but neovascularization is also likely to develop in future.
If exudation is localized mainly around the macula, where it often forms large
deposits, the disturbance of circulation is very likely confined to the capillary network
around the posterior pole. The progression of exudation may remain restricted to
this area of the fundus for a period of years. In these cases neovascularization
is not likely to develop but visual deterioration will be very marked.

c Neovascularization

If networks of dilated and hypertrophic capillary loops appear at various sites in
the mid periphery of the fundus and numerous cotton-wool spots, beading of the
veins and narrowing of the small arterial branches are present, a severe disturbance
of the retinal circulation is to be assumed. A progression of neovascularization
is very likely to occur and the appearance of large networks of newly-formed vessels
on the surface of the retina is to be expected (case of figure 16).

If neovascularization networks are already developed, and marked beading of the
veins and occluded arterial branches are present, a very severe disturbance of the
retinal circulation is to be assumed. A further rapid deterioration of the circulation
with deviation of the blood stream to the growing networks of newly-formed vessels
and simultaneous occlusion of retinal arterioles is to be expected. If at the same
time retraction of the posterior vitreous membrane is observed, massive preretinal
haemorrhages are likely to occur in a short time (cases of figure 19 and figure 25).
When neovascularization is restricted to the disc, the fundus often presents a very
moderate retinopathy. If at the same time the small arterial branches are narrowed
and of irregular calibre a very severe disturbance of the circulation may be assumed

not only in the retinal vascular tree but in the ciliary vascular system as well.
Rubeosis of the iris and haemorrhagic glaucoma are very likely to develop.

d Fibrous proliferation

In case fibrous proliferation is associated with large networks of newly-formed
vessels on the surface of the retina and the fibrous strands are adherent to a
retracting posterior vitreous membrane, this situation may lead at short notice to
massive vitreous haemorrhage, retinal schisis or retinal detachment (case of fig. 28).
However, if during the development of detachment retinal holes have not formed,
the detachment may remain confined to a part of the fundus only. If fibrous
proliferation is not associated with vitreous retraction the condition may remain
unchanged for many years (case of fig. 24).
A long-term stabilization of the clinical picture may happen too if the fibrous strands
are attached only to the disc and the newly-formed vessels within the strands
have obliterated before haemorrhages occur. In this case the pulling effect of the
retracting posterior vitreous membrane on the prepapillary avascular fibrous tissue
is no longer to be feared.

Effect of photocoagulation

If progression of the disease and deterioration of vision is to be expected, treatment
with photocoagulation should be considered. The probable effect of photocoagulation
upon the different symptoms has been shown in the preceding series of fundus
photographs. We must stress that these examples cannot cover the whole range
of possible postcoagulative evolutions. However, they provide evidence of what
can be achieved by photocoagulation. Some pathological changes may diminish
or even disappear after treatment. Others may remain unchanged or even progress
despite of, or as some say, because of photocoagulation.

Intraretinal haemorrhages and microaneurysms disappear within a few months.
The engorgement of the veins may improve as well.
The same holds for the retinal edema, often found in the vicinity of fatty exudates;
edema of the retina is drained away before the fatty exudates disappear. The cystic
edema of the macula is however refractory and does not respond to photocoagulation.

Small fatty exudates and small newly-formed vessels usually need more than 3
months to vanish, while larger networks of newly-formed vessels, even a year
after treatment, may still be present though reduced in size.
Preretinal haemorrhages disappear and do not recur if the source can be adequately
treated. However, if the bleeding vessel is pulled away from the surface of the
retina, coagulation may be difficult or even impossible.
The improvement or, eventually, the stabilization of the clinical picture of diabetic
retinopathy depends mainly upon the condition of the small arterial branches of
the retinal vascular network. The influence of photocoagulation is unsufficient or
lacking in those cases in which the arterial supply is irreversibly disturbed owing
to wide-spread narrowing and occlusion of the small arterial branches.

The rationale of photocoagulation

In treating diabetic retinopathy, we coagulate all pathological changes we can
see ophthalmoscopically or that we can detect by means of additional fluorography.
In this way leaking parts of the capillary network, newly-formed vessels and retinal
tissue, at the site of these pathological changes, are destroyed. As a consequence
of this treatment a great number of scars and numerous areas of destroyed capillaries
are produced. Following treatment the fundus picture may show an appearance
which one is inclined to call 'quiet'. The retinal veins are no longer engorged
and the retina looks 'dry' and 'clean'.
This overall improvement of the clinical picture has generally been attributed to
the destruction of retinal tissue. The scarring of the hypoxic areas of the retina
is assumed to restore a previously disturbed balance between oxygen need and
oxygen supply, and consequently to prevent the production of a hypothetic
vasoformative factor.
In our opinion, a more plausible explanation may be that improvement is due
essentially to the destruction of the pathological parts of the capillary network.
We assume that diabetic retinopathy is basically due to a decompensation of the
retinal circulation. On the one hand there is a dense capillary network with thickned
vessel walls, and on the other an insufficient arterial supply and probably an equally
insufficient venous drainage. The result is stagnation of blood flow, ectatic changes
of the capillary walls, areas of leakage and capillary closure. The following sequence
of events are also due basically to disturbed circulation. They start with dilatation
and hypertrophy of the capillaries adjacent to the nonperfused zones and end with
large networks of newly-formed vessels. Most of the pathological changes are
found at those sites of the retinal vascular tree, at which haemodynamics meet
difficulties. This provides further support for the assumption that the main cause
of diabetic retinopathy is of a haemodynamic nature.
By means of photocoagulation, the pathological parts of the capillary network and
the newly-formed vessels are destroyed. This leads not only to the removal of
changes causing exudation and haemorrhages, but also reduces the whole volume
of the capillary bed, readapting it to the reduced arterial supply. At the same time
the blood flow is forced to keep to the still more or less normal part of the retinal
vascular network.

Extensive 'ablative' photocoagulation of healthy looking parts of the fundus has
been proven to be beneficial in cases with neovascularization on the disc (7, 8,
9, 18).
In our experience treatment may be beneficial even if restricted to the sites with
unfavourable haemodynamic circumstances such as the areas around the
arterio-venous crossings and the stripes along the retinal veins. In this way we
may be able to achieve the same result avoiding unnecessary destruction of retinal
tissue.
When treating diabetic retinopathy by photocoagulation, we should be permanently
aware of the need to balance the ills we cure against the ills we cause.

References

1 Oakley, N. W. et al. Diabetic retinopathy. I. The assessment of severity and progress by comparison with a set of standard fundus photographs. Diabetologia 3: 402 (1967).

2 Davis, M. D., E. W. D. Norton & F. L. Myers. Airlie classification of diabetic retinopathy. In: Symposium on the treatment of diabetic retinopathy, p. 7; ed. by M. F. Goldberg and S. L. Fine. U.S. Department of Health, Education and Welfare, Virginia, 1968.

3 Zweng, H. C., H. L. Little & R. R. Peabody. Argon laser photocoagulation of diabetic retinopathy. Arch. Ophthal. 86: 395 (1971).

4 Little, H. L. & H. C. Zweng. Photocoagulation au laser à l'Argon dans les affections maculaires et les rétinopathies diabétiques. Arch. Ophtal. 32: 789 (1972).

5 Little, H. L. & H. C. Zweng. Paper, read at the 'Laser-meeting' in Albi on 22 May 1974.

6 L'Esperance, F. A. Argon laser photocoagulation of diabetic retinal neovascularization (a five-year appraisal). Trans. Amer. Acad. Ophthal. Otolaryng. 77: 6 (1973).

7 Aiello, L. M. et al. Ruby laser photocoagulation in treatment of diabetic proliferating retinopathy: preliminary report. In: Symposium on the treatment of diabetic retinopathy, p. 437; ed. by M. F. Goldberg and S. L. Fine. U.S. Department of Health, Education and Welfare, Virginia, 1968.

8 Okun, E. & G. P. Johnston. Role of photocoagulation in the treatment of proliferative diabetic retinopathy; continuation and follow-up studies. In: Symposium on the treatment of diabetic retinopathy, p. 523; ed. by M. F. Goldberg and S. L. Fine. U.S. Department of Health, Education and Welfare, Virginia, 1968.

9 Taylor, E. Proliferative diabetic retinopathy. Brit. J. Ophthal. 54: 535 (1970).

10 Behrendt, T. Therapeutic vascular occlusions in diabetic retinopathy. Arch. Ophthal. 87: 629 (1972).

11 Riaskoff, S. Die diabetische Retinopathie und ihre Behandlung mit Lichtkoagulation. Docum. Ophthal. 32: 225 (1972).

12 Riaskoff, S. Treatment of diabetic retinopathy with light coagulation. Trans. Ophthal. Soc. U.K. 92: 835 (1972).

13 Meyer-Schwickerath, G. R. E. & A. Wessing. Fluorescein study in cases of diabetic retinopathy treated with photocoagulation. Proc. Int. Symp. Fluorescein Angiography, Albi 1969, p. 400. Karger, Basel, 1971.

14 Cheng, H., Blach, R. K., Hamilton, A. M. & E. M. Kohner. Diabetic maculopathy. Trans. Ophthal. Soc. U.K. 92: 407 (1972).

15 Patz, A., H. Schatz, J. W. Berkow, A. M. Gittelson & U. Ticho. Macular edema — an overlooked complication of diabetic retinopathy. Trans. Amer. Acad. Ophthal. Otolaryng. 77: 34 (1973).

16 Riaskoff, S. Die Bedeutung der Lichtkoagulation für die Behandlung der diabetischen Retinopathie des alternden Diabetikers. Z. Geront. 6: 17 (1973).

17 Rubinstein, K. & V. Myska. Pathogenesis and treatment of diabetic maculopathy. Brit. J. Ophthal. 58: 76 (1974).

18 Wessing, A. K. & Meyer-Schwickerath, G R E. Results of photocoagulation in diabetic retinopathy. In Goldberg, M. F. and Fine, S. L. (eds.) Symposium on treatment of diabetic retinopathy. Arlington, Va., U.S. Dept. Health, Education and Welfare, pp. 569–592 (1968).